SWINE FLU
Diagnosis and Treatment

SWINE FLU
Diagnosis and Treatment

by
Sameer Prakash

BIOTECH

2010
Biotech Books
Delhi - 110 035

ISBN 81-7622-168-6
ISBN 978-81-7622-168-9

Published by : **BIOTECH BOOKS**
1123/74, Tri Nagar,
Delhi - 110 035
Phone: 27383999
e-mail: biotechbooks@yahoo.co.in

Showroom : 4762-63/23, Ansari Road, Darya Ganj,
New Delhi - 110 002
Phone: 23245578, 23244987

Printed at : **Chawla Offset Printers**
New Delhi - 110 052

PRINTED IN INDIA

Preface

Swine flu, also known as Swine influenza (also called hog flu, and pig flu) is an infection of a host animal by any one of several specific types of microscopic organisms, called "swine influenza virus".

In 2009, the media labelled as "swine flu", the flu caused by 2009's new strain of swine-origin A/H1N1 pandemic virus. A swine influenza virus (SIV) is an strain of the influenza family of viruses that is usually hosted by pigs. As of 2009, the known SIV strains are the influenza C virus and the subtypes of the influenza A virus, known as H1N1, H1N2, H3N1, H3N2, and H2N3. Swine influenza is common in pigs in United States (particularly in the midwest and occasionally in other areas), Mexico, Canada, South America, Europe (including United Kingdom, Sweden and Italy), Kenya, and Eastern Asia (mainly China, Taiwan, and Japan).

Transmission of swine influenza virus from pigs to humans is not common and does not always cause human influenza, often only resulting in the production of antibodies in blood. The meat of the animal poses no risk of transmitting the virus, when properly cooked. If transmission does cause human influenza, it is called zoonotic swine flu. People, who work with pigs, especially people with intense exposures, are at increased risk of catching swine flu. In mid-20th century, identification of influenza subtypes became possible, which allowed accurate diagnosis of transmission to humans. Since then, fifty confirmed transmissions have been recorded, Rarely, these strains of swine flu can pass from human to human. In humans, the symptoms of swine flu are similar to those of influenza and of influenza-like illness in general, namely chill, fever, sore throat, muscle pain, severe headache, coughing, weakness and general discomfort.

The 2009 swine flu outbreak in humans, was due to a new strain of influenza A virus subtype H1N1 that contains genes, is closely related to swine influenza. The origin of this new strain is unknown. However, the World Organisation for Animal Health reports that this strain has not been isolated in pigs. This strain can be transmitted from human to human and causes the normal symptoms of influenza. Pigs can also become infected with human influenza, and this appears to have happened, during the 1918 flu pandemic and again in 2009 swine flu outbreak.

Swine Flu is a new subject of study and perhaps, so far, there is no significant book on it. Hence, this meticulous effort, for presenting a comprehensive, exhaustive and to a maximum extent, an authentic work. This research-based book is bound to receive due appreciation and warm welcome in all concerned circles. Enlightening comments are eagerly invited from wise readers.

— ***Sameer Prakash***

Contents

1

Introduction

Swine Flu (also called swine influenza, hog flu, and pig flu) is an infection of a host animal by any one of several specific types of microscopic organisms called "swine influenza virus". A swine influenza virus (SIV) is any strain of the influenza family of viruses that is usually hosted by (is endemic in) pigs. As of 2009, the known SIV strains are the influenza C virus and the subtypes of the influenza A virus known as H1N1, H1N2, H3N1, H3N2, and H2N3. Swine influenza is common in pigs in the midwestern United States (and occasionally in other states), Mexico, Canada, South America, Europe (including the United Kingdom, Sweden, and Italy), Kenya, Mainland China, Taiwan, Japan and other parts of eastern Asia.

Transmission of swine influenza virus from pigs to humans is not common and does not always cause human influenza, often only resulting in the production of antibodies in the blood. The meat of the animal poses no risk of transmitting the virus when properly cooked. If transmission does cause human influenza, it is called zoonotic swine flu. People who work with pigs, especially people with intense exposures, are at increased risk of catching swine flu. In the mid-20th century, identification of influenza subtypes became possible, this allows accurate diagnosis of transmission to humans. Since then, fifty confirmed transmissions have been recorded, Rarely, these strains of swine flu can pass from human to human. In humans, the symptoms of swine flu are similar to those of influenza and of influenza-like illness in general, namely chills, fever, sore throat, muscle pains, severe headache, coughing, weakness and general discomfort.

The 2009 swine flu outbreak in humans is due to a new strain of influenza A virus subtype H1N1 that contains genes closely related to swine influenza. The origin of this new strain is unknown. However, the World Organisation for Animal Health (OIE) reports that this strain has not been isolated in pigs. This strain can be transmitted from human to human, and causes the normal symptoms of influenza.

Pigs can become infected with human influenza, and this appears to have happened during the 1918 flu pandemic and the 2009 swine flu outbreak.

The Backdrop

Swine influenza was first proposed to be a disease related to human influenza during the 1918 flu pandemic, when pigs became sick at the same time as humans. The first identification of an influenza virus as a cause of disease in pigs occurred about ten years later, in 1930. For the following 60 years, swine influenza strains were almost exclusively H1N1. Then, between 1997 and 2002, new strains of three different subtypes and five different genotypes emerged as causes of influenza among pigs in North America. In 1997-1998, H3N2 strains emerged. These strains, which include genes derived by reassortment from human, swine and avian viruses, have become a major cause of swine influenza in North America. Reassortment between H1N1 and H3N2 produced H1N2. In 1999 in Canada, a strain of H4N6 crossed the species barrier from birds to pigs, but was contained on a single farm.

The H1N1 form of swine flu is one of the descendants of the strain that caused the 1918 flu pandemic. As well as persisting in pigs, the descendants of the 1918 virus have also circulated in humans through the 20th century, contributing to the normal seasonal epidemics of influenza. However, direct transmission from pigs to humans is rare, with only 12 cases in the US since 2005. Nevertheless, the retention of influenza strains in pigs after these strains have disappeared from the human population might make pigs a reservoir where influenza viruses could persist, later emerging to reinfect humans once human immunity to these strains has waned.

Swine flu has been reported numerous times as a zoonosis in humans, usually with limited distribution, rarely with a widespread distribution. Outbreaks in swine are common and cause significant economic losses in industry, primarily by causing stunting and extended time to market. For example, this disease costs the British meat industry about £65 million every year.

Signs and Symptoms

In Swine

In pigs influenza infection produces fever, lethargy, sneezing, coughing, difficulty breathing and decreased appetite. In some cases the infection can cause abortion. Although mortality is usually low (around 1-4%), the virus can produce weight loss and poor growth, causing economic loss to farmers. Infected pigs can lose up to 12 pounds of body weight over a 3 to 4 week period.

In Humans

Direct transmission of a swine flu virus from pigs to humans is occasionally possible (called zoonotic swine flu). In all, 50 cases are known to have occurred since the first report in medical literature in 1958, which have resulted in a total of six deaths. Of these six people, one was pregnant, one had leukaemia, one had Hodgkin disease and two were known to be previously healthy. Despite these apparently low numbers of infections, the true rate of infection may be higher, since most cases only cause a very mild disease, and will probably never be reported or diagnosed. According to the Centres for Disease Control and Prevention (CDC), in humans the symptoms of the 2009 "swine flu" H1N1 virus are similar to those of influenza and of influenza-like illness in general.

Symptoms include fever, cough, sore throat, body aches, headache, chills and fatigue. The 2009 outbreak has shown an increased percentage of patients reporting diarrhoea and vomiting. The 2009 H1N1 virus is not zoonotic swine flu, as it is not transmitted from pigs to humans, but from person to person.

Because these symptoms are not specific to swine flu, a differential diagnosis of *probable* swine flu requires not only symptoms but also a high likelihood of swine flu due to the person's recent history. For example, during the 2009 swine flu outbreak in the United States, CDC advised physicians to "consider swine influenza infection in the differential diagnosis of patients with acute febrile respiratory illness who have either been in contact with persons with confirmed swine flu, or who were in one of the five US states that have reported swine flu cases or in Mexico during the 7 days preceding their illness onset." A diagnosis of *confirmed* swine flu requires laboratory testing of a respiratory sample (a simple nose and throat swab).

Classification

H3N2 is a subtype of the viral genus Influenza virus A, which is an important cause of human influenza. Its name derives from the forms of the two kinds of proteins on the surface of its coat, hemagglutinin (H) and neuraminidase (N). By reassortment, H3N2 exchanges genes for internal proteins with other influenza subtypes.

Seasonal H3N2 Flu

Seasonal influenza kills an estimated 36,000 people in the United States each year. Flu vaccines are based on predicting which mutants of H1N1, H3N2, H1N2, and influenza B will proliferate in the next season. Separate vaccines are developed for the northern and southern hemispheres in preparation for their annual epidemics. In the tropics, influenza shows no clear seasonality. In the past ten years, H3N2 has tended to dominate in prevalence over H1N1, H1N2, and influenza B. Measured resistance to the standard antiviral drugs amantadine and rimantadine in H3N2 has increased from 1 per cent in 1994 to 12 per cent in 2003 to 91 per cent in 2005.

Seasonal H3N2 flu is a human flu from H3N2 that is slightly different from one of last year's flu season H3N2 variants. Seasonal influenza viruses flow out of overlapping epidemics in East and South East Asia, then trickle around the globe before dying off. Identifying the source of the viruses allows global health officials to better predict which viruses are most likely to cause the most disease over the next year. An analysis of 13,000 samples of influenza A/H3N2 virus that were collected across six continents from 2002 to 2007 by the WHO's Global Influenza Surveillance Network showed that newly emerging strains of H3N2 appeared in East and South East Asian countries about 6 to 9 months earlier than anywhere else. The strains generally reached Australia and New Zealand next, followed by North America and Europe. The new variants typically reached South America after an additional 6 to 9 months, the group reported.

The Virus

> "In swine, 3 influenza A virus subtypes (H1N1, H3N2, and H1N2) are circulating throughout the world. In the United States, the classic H1N1 subtype was exclusively prevalent among swine populations before 1998; however, since late-August 1998, H3N2 subtypes have been isolated from pigs. Most H3N2 virus isolates are triple reassortants, containing genes from human (HA, NA, and PB1), swine (NS, NP, and M), and avian (PB2 and PA) lineages. [...] Present vaccination strategies for SIV control and prevention in swine farms typically include the use of 1 of several bivalent SIV vaccines commercially available in the United States. Of the 97 recent H3N2 isolates examined, only 41 isolates had strong serologic cross-reactions with antiserum to 3 commercial SIV

> vaccines. Since the protective ability of influenza vaccines depends primarily on the closeness of the match between the vaccine virus and the epidemic virus, the presence of non-reactive H3N2 SIV variants suggests that current commercial vaccines might not effectively protect pigs from infection with a majority of H3N2 viruses."

Avian influenza virus H3N2 is endemic in pigs in China and has been detected in pigs in Vietnam, increasing fears of the emergence of new variant strains. Health experts say pigs can carry human influenza viruses, which can combine (i.e. exchange homologous genome sub-units by genetic reassortment) with H5N1, passing genes and mutating into a form which can pass easily among humans. H3N2 evolved from H2N2 by antigenic shift and caused the Hong Kong Flu pandemic of 1968 and 1969 that killed up to 750,000 humans. The dominant strain of annual flu in humans in January 2006 is H3N2. Measured resistance to the standard antiviral drugs amantadine and rimantadine in H3N2 in humans has increased to 91 per cent in 2005. In August 2004, researchers in China found H5N1 in pigs.

Mortality

The global mortality rate from the 1918/1919 pandemic is not known, but it is estimated that 10 per cent to 20 per cent of those who were infected died. With about a third of the world population infected, this case-fatality ratio means that 3 per cent to 6 per cent of the entire global population died. Influenza may have killed as many as 25 million in its first 25 weeks. Older estimates say it killed 40–50 million people while current estimates say 50 million to 100 million people worldwide were killed. This pandemic has been described as "the greatest medical holocaust in history" and may have killed more people than the Black Death.

As many as 17 million died in India, about 5 per cent of India's population at the time. In Japan, 23 million persons were affected, and 390,000 died. In the US, about 28 per cent of the population suffered, and 500,000 to 675,000 died. In Britain as many as 250,000 died; in France more than 400,000. In Canada approximately 50,000 died. Entire villages perished in Alaska and southern Africa. Ras Tafari (the future Haile Selassie) was one of the first Ethiopians who contracted influenza but survived, although many of his subjects did not; estimates for the fatalities in the capital city, Addis Ababa, range from 5,000 to 10,000, with some experts opining that the number was even higher, while in British Somaliland one official there estimated that 7 per cent of the native population died from influenza. In Australia an estimated 12,000 people died and in the Fiji Islands, 14 per cent of the population died during only two weeks, and in Western Samoa 22 per cent.

This huge death toll was caused by an extremely high infection rate of up to 50 per cent and the extreme severity of the symptoms, suspected to be caused by cytokine storms. Indeed, symptoms in 1918 were so unusual that initially influenza was misdiagnosed as dengue, cholera, or typhoid. One observer wrote, "One of the most striking of the complications was haemorrhage from mucous membranes, especially from the nose, stomach, and intestine. Bleeding from the ears and petechial haemorrhages in the skin also occurred." The majority of deaths were from bacterial pneumonia, a secondary infection caused by influenza, but the virus also killed people directly, causing massive haemorrhages and edema in the lung.

Origin of the Name

Although the first cases of the disease were registered in the continental US and the rest of Europe long before getting to Spain, the 1918 Flu received its nickname "Spanish Flu" because Spain, a neutral country in WW I, had no special censorship for news against the disease and its consequences. Hence the most reliable news came from Spain, giving the false impression that Spain was the most—if not the only—affected zone.

History: While World War I did not cause the flu, the close troop quarters and massive troop movements hastened the pandemic, and increased transmission augmented mutation and may have increased the lethality of the virus. Some researchers speculate that the soldiers' immune systems were weakened by malnourishment, and the stresses of combat and chemical attacks, increasing their susceptibility to the disease. Price-Smith has made the controversial argument that the virus helped tip the balance of power in the latter days of the war towards the Allied cause. Specifically, he provides data that the viral waves hit the Central Powers before they hit the Allied powers, and that both morbidity and mortality in Germany and Austria were considerably higher than in Britain and France.

A large factor of worldwide flu occurrence was increased travel. Modern transportation systems made it easier for soldiers, sailors, and civilian travellers to spread the disease quickly to communities worldwide.

Geographic Sources

Some scholars have theorised that the flu probably originated in the Far East. Dr. C. Hannoun, leading expert of the 1918 flu for the Institute Pasteur noticed that the former virus was likely to have come from China, mutated in the United States near Boston, and spread to Brest (France), Europe's battlefields, Europe, and the world using Allied soldiers and sailors as main spreaders. C. Hannoun also designated several other theories, such as Spain, Kansas, and Brest, as being possible but not likely.

Historian Alfred W. Crosby observed that the flu seems to have originated in Kansas. Political scientist Andrew Price-Smith published data from the Austrian archives suggesting that the influenza had earlier origins, beginning in Austria in the spring of 1917. Popular writer John Barry echoed Crosby in proposing that Haskell County, Kansas was the location of the first outbreak of flu. In the United States the disease was first observed at Fort Riley, Kansas, United States, on March 4, 1918, and Queens, New York, on March 11, 1918. In August 1918, a more virulent strain appeared simultaneously in Brest, France, in Freetown, Sierra Leone, and in the US at Boston, Massachusetts. The Allies of World War I came to call it the Spanish flu, primarily because the pandemic received greater press attention after it moved from France to Spain in November 1918. Spain was not involved in the war and had not imposed wartime censorship.

Investigative work by a British team, led by virologist John Oxford of St. Bartholomew's Hospital and the Royal London Hospital, has suggested that a principal British troop staging camp in Étaples, France was at the centre of the 1918 flu pandemic, or was the location of a significant precursor virus.

Patterns of Fatality

The influenza strain was unusual in that this pandemic killed many young adults and otherwise healthy victims; typical influenzas kill mostly weak individuals, such as infants (aged 0-2 years), the elderly, and the immunocompromised. Older adults may have had some immunity from the earlier Russian flu pandemic of 1889. Another oddity was that the outbreak was widespread in summer and fall (in the Northern Hemisphere); influenza is usually worse in winter.

In fast-progressing cases, mortality was primarily from pneumonia, by virus-induced pulmonary consolidation. Slower-progressing cases featured secondary bacterial pneumonias, and there may have been neural involvement that led to mental disorders in some cases. Some deaths resulted from malnourishment and even animal attacks in overwhelmed communities.

Deadly Second Wave

The second wave of the 1918 pandemic was much deadlier than the first. During the first wave, which began in early-March, the epidemic resembled typical flu epidemics. Those at the most risk were the sick and elderly, and younger, healthier people recovered easily. But in August, when the second wave began in France, Sierra Leone and the United States, the virus had mutated to a much more deadly form. This has been attributed to the circumstances of the first World War. In civilian life evolutionary pressures favour a mild strain: those who get really sick stay home, but those mildly ill continue with their lives, go to work and go shopping, preferentially spreading the mild strain.

In the trenches the evolutionary pressures were reversed: soldiers with a mild strain remained where they were, while the severely ill were sent on crowded trains to crowded field hospitals, spreading the deadlier virus. So the second wave began and flu quickly spread around the world again. It was the same flu, in that those who recovered from first-wave infections were immune, but it was far more deadly, and the most vulnerable people were those like the soldiers in the trenches—young, otherwise healthy, adults. Consequently, during modern pandemics, health officials pay attention when the virus reaches places with social upheaval, looking for deadlier strains of the virus.

Devastated Communities

Even in areas where mortality was low, so many people were incapacitated that much of everyday life stopped. Some communities closed all stores or required customers to leave their orders outside the store. There were many reports of places where the health-care workers could not tend the sick nor the grave-diggers bury the dead because they too were ill. Mass graves were dug by steam shovel and bodies buried without coffins in many places. Several Pacific island territories were particularly hard-hit. The pandemic reached them from New Zealand, which was too slow to implement measures to prevent ships carrying the flu from leaving its ports. From New Zealand the flu reached Tonga (killing 8 per cent of the population), Nauru (16%) and Fiji (5 per cent, 9000 people).

Worst affected was Western Samoa, a territory then under New Zealand military administration. A crippling 90 per cent of the population was infected; 30 per cent of adult men, 22 per cent of adult women and 10 per cent of children were killed. By contrast, the flu was kept away from American Samoa by a commander who imposed a blockade. The mortality rate in New Zealand itself was 5 per cent.

Less Affected Areas

In Japan, 257,363 deaths were attributed to influenza by July 1919, giving an estimated 0.425 per cent mortality rate, much lower than nearly all other Asian countries for which data are available. The Japanese government severely restricted maritime travel to and from the home islands when the pandemic struck.

In the Pacific, American Samoa and the French colony of New Caledonia also succeeded in preventing even a single death from influenza through effective quarantines. In Australia, nearly 12,000 perished.

End of the Pandemic

After the lethal second wave struck in the fall of 1918, the disease died down abruptly. New cases almost dropped to nothing after the peak in the second wave. In Philadelphia for example, 4,597 people died in the week ending October 16, but by November 11 influenza had almost disappeared from the city. One explanation for the rapid decline of the lethality of the disease is that doctors simply got better at preventing and treating the pneumonia which developed after the victims had contracted the virus, although John Barry states in his book that researchers have found no evidence to support this. Another theory holds that the 1918 virus mutated extremely rapidly to a less lethal strain. This is a common occurrence with influenza viruses: there is a general tendency for pathogenic viruses to become less lethal as time goes by, providing more living hosts. According to this theory, this happened very quickly for the 1918 virus.

Cultural Impact

In the United States, Great Britain and other countries, despite the relatively high morbidity and mortality rates that resulted from the epidemic in 1918-1919, the Spanish flu began to fade from public awareness over the decades until the arrival of news about bird flu and other pandemics in the 1990s and 2000s. This has led some historians to label the Spanish flu a "forgotten pandemic." One of the only major works of American literature written after 1918 that deals directly with the Spanish flu is Katherine Anne Porter's *Pale Horse, Pale Rider*. In 1935 John O'Hara wrote a long short story, "The Doctor's Son," about the experience of his fictional alter ego during the flu epidemic in a Pennsylvania coal mining town. In 1937 American novelist William Keepers Maxwell, Jr. wrote *They Came Like Swallows*, a fictional reconstruction of the events surrounding his mother's death from the flu. Mary McCarthy, the American novelist and essayist, wrote about her parents' deaths in *Memories of a Catholic Girlhood*. In 1992 Bodie and Brock Thoene's "Shiloh Legacy" series leads off with an account of the Spanish Flu in New York and Arkansas in their fictional novel *In My Father's House*. In 1997 David Morrell's short story If I Die Before I Wake — dealing with a small American town during the second wave — was published in the anthology REVELATIONS, which was framed by Clive Barker. In 2006 Thomas Mullen wrote a novel called *The Last Town on Earth* about the impact of the Spanish flu on a fictional mill town in Washington.

Several theories have been offered as to why the Spanish flu may have been "forgotten" by historians and the public over so many years. These include the rapid pace of the pandemic (it killed most of its victims in the United States, for example, within a period of less than nine months), previous familiarity with pandemic disease in the late-19th and early-20th centuries, and the distraction of the First World War.

Another explanation involves the age group affected by the disease. The majority of fatalities, in both World War I and in the Spanish Flu epidemic, were young adults. The deaths caused by the flu may have been overlooked due to the large numbers of deaths of young men in the war or as a result of injuries. When people read the obituaries of the era, they saw the war or post-war deaths and the deaths from the influenza side by side. Particularly in Europe, where the war's toll was extremely high, the flu may not have had a great, separate, psychological impact, or may have seemed a mere "extension" of the war's tragedies.

The duration of the pandemic and the war could also play a role: the disease would usually only affect a certain area for a month before leaving, while the war, which most expected to end quickly, had lasted for four years by the time the pandemic struck. This left little time for the disease to have a significant impact on the economy. During this time period pandemic outbreaks were not uncommon: typhoid, yellow fever, diphtheria, and cholera all occurred near the same time period. These outbreaks probably lessened the significance of the influenza pandemic for the public.

Pandemic in Humans 1918

The 1918 flu pandemic in humans was associated with H1N1 and influenza appearing in pigs, this may reflect a zoonosis either from swine to humans, or from humans to swine. Although it is not certain in which direction the virus was transferred, some evidence suggests that, in this case, pigs caught the disease from humans. For instance, swine influenza was only noted as a new disease of pigs in 1918, after the first large outbreaks of influenza amongst people. Although a recent phylogenetic analysis of more recent strains of influenza in humans, birds, and swine suggests that the 1918 outbreak in humans followed a reassortment event within a mammal, the exact origin of the 1918 strain remains elusive.

Hong Kong Flu 1968-1969

The Hong Kong Flu was a category 2 flu pandemic caused by a strain of H3N2 descended from H2N2 by antigenic shift, in which genes from multiple subtypes reassorted to form a new virus. This pandemic of 1968 and 1969 killed an estimated one million people worldwide. The pandemic infected an estimated 500,000 Hong Kong residents, 15 per cent of the population, with a low death rate. In the United States, approximately 33,800 people died.

Both the H2N2 and H3N2 pandemic flu strains contained genes from avian influenza viruses. The new subtypes arose in pigs coinfected with avian and human viruses and were soon transferred to humans. Swine were considered the original "intermediate host" for influenza, because they supported reassortment of divergent subtypes. However, other hosts appear capable of similar coinfection (e.g., many poultry species), and direct transmission of avian viruses to humans is possible. H1N1 may have been transmitted directly from birds to humans (Belshe 2005).

The Hong Kong flu strain shared internal genes and the neuraminidase with the 1957 Asian Flu (H2N2). Accumulated antibodies to the neuraminidase or internal proteins may have resulted in much fewer casualties than most pandemics. However, cross-immunity within and between subtypes of influenza is poorly understood.

The Hong Kong flu was the first known outbreak of the H3N2 strain, though there is serologic evidence of H3N2 infections in the late-19th century. The first record of the outbreak in Hong Kong appeared on 13 July 1968 in an area with a density of about 500 people per acre in an urban setting. The outbreak reached maximum intensity in 2 weeks, lasting 6 weeks in total. The virus was isolated in Queen Mary Hospital. Flu symptoms lasted 4 to 5 days.

By July 1968, extensive outbreaks were reported in Vietnam and Singapore. By September 1968, it reached India, Philippines, northern Australia and Europe. That same month, the virus entered California from returning Vietnam War troops. It would reach Japan, Africa and South America by 1969.

> "Three strains of Hong Kong influenza virus isolated from humans were compared with a strain

> isolated from a calf for their ability to cause disease in calves. One of the human strains. A/Aichi/2/68, was detected for five days in a calf, but all three failed to cause signs of disease. Strain A/cal/Duschanbe/55/71 could be detected for seven days and caused an influenza-like illness in calves."

Outbreak in USA 1976

On February 5, 1976, in the United States an army recruit at Fort Dix said he felt tired and weak. He died the next day and four of his fellow soldiers were later hospitalised. Two weeks after his death, health officials announced that the cause of death was a new strain of swine flu. The strain, a variant of H1N1, is known as A/New Jersey/1976 (H1N1). It was detected only from January 19 to February 9 and did not spread beyond Fort Dix.

This new strain appeared to be closely related to the strain involved in the 1918 flu pandemic. Moreover, the ensuing increased surveillance uncovered another strain in circulation in the US: A/Victoria/75 (H3N2) spread simultaneously, also caused illness, and persisted until March. Alarmed public-health officials decided action must be taken to head off another major pandemic, and urged President Gerald Ford that every person in the US be vaccinated for the disease.

The vaccination programme was plagued by delays and public relations problems. On October 1, 1976, the immunisation programme began and by October 11, approximately 40 million people, or about 24 per cent of the population, had received swine flu immunisations. That same day, three senior citizens died soon after receiving their swine flu shots and there was a media outcry linking the deaths to the immunisations, despite the lack of positive proof. According to science writer Patrick Di Justo, however, by the time the truth was known — that the deaths were not proven to be related to the vaccine — it was too late. "The government had long feared mass panic about swine flu — now they feared mass panic about the swine flu vaccinations." This became a strong setback to the programme.

There were reports of Guillain-Barré syndrome, a paralysing neuromuscular disorder, affecting some people who had received swine flu immunisations. This syndrome is a rare side-effect of modern influenza vaccines, with an incidence of about one case per million vaccinations. As a result, Di Justo writes that "the public refused to trust a government-operated health programme that killed old people and crippled young people." In total, less than 33 per cent of the population had been immunised by the end of 1976. The National Influenza Immunisation Programme was effectively halted on Dec. 16.

Overall, there were about 500 cases of Guillain-Barré syndrome (GBS), resulting in death from severe pulmonary complications for 25 people, which, according to Dr. P. Haber, were probably caused by an immunopathological reaction to the 1976 vaccine. Other influenza vaccines have not been linked to GBS, though caution is advised for certain individuals, particularly those with a history of GBS. Still, as observed by a participant in the immunisation programme, the vaccine killed more Americans than the disease did.

Zoonosis 1988

In September 1988, a swine flu virus killed one woman and infected others. 32-year-old Barbara Ann Wieners was eight months pregnant when she and her husband, Ed, became ill after visiting the hog barn at a county fair in Walworth County, Wisconsin. Barbara died eight days later, after developing pneumonia. The only pathogen identified was an H1N1 strain of swine influenza virus. Doctors were able to induce labour and deliver a healthy daughter before she died. Her husband recovered from his symptoms.

ILI was reportedly widespread among the pigs exhibited at the fair. 76 per cent of 25 swine exhibitors aged 9 to 19 tested positive for antibody to SIV, but no serious illnesses were detected among this group. Additional studies suggested between one and three health care personnel who had contact with the patient developed mild influenza-like illnesses with antibody evidence of swine flu infection. However, there was no community outbreak.

Outbreak of Swine in USA 1998

In 1998, swine flu was found in pigs in four US states. Within a year, it had spread through pig populations across the United States. Scientists found that this virus had originated in pigs as a recombinant form of flu strains from birds and humans. This outbreak confirmed that pigs can serve as a crucible where novel influenza viruses emerge as a result of the reassortment of genes from different strains.

Fujian Flu 2003-2004

Fujian flu refers to flu caused by either a Fujian human flu strain of the H3N2 subtype of the *Influenza A virus* or a Fujian bird flu strain of the H5N1 subtype of the *Influenza A virus.* These strains are named after Fujian, a coastal province of the People's Republic of China that is across the Taiwan strait from Taiwan.

A/Fujian (H3N2) human flu [from A/Fujian/411/2002(H3N2) -like flu virus strains] caused an unusually severe 2003–2004 flu season. This was due to a reassortment event that caused a minor clade to provide a haemagglutinin gene that later became part of the dominant strain in the 2002-2003 flu season. A/Fujian (H3N2) was made part of the trivalent influenza vaccine for the 2004–2005 flu season and its descendants are still the most common human H3N2 strain.

Flu Season 2004–2005

The 2004–05 trivalent influenza vaccine for the United States contained A/New Caledonia/20/99-like (H1N1), A/Fujian/411/2002-like (H3N2), and B/Shanghai/361/2002-like viruses.

Flu Season 2005–2006

The vaccines produced for the 2005–2006 season use:

- an A/New Caledonia/20/1999-like(H1N1);
- an A/California/7/2004-like(H3N2) (or the antigenically equivalent strain A/New York/55/2004);
- a B/Jiangsu/10/2003-like viruses.

Flu Season 2006–2007

The 2006–2007 influenza vaccine composition recommended by the World Health Organisation on 15 February 2006 and the US FDA's Vaccines and Related Biological Products Advisory Committee (VRBPAC) on 17 February 2006 use:

- an A/New Caledonia/20/99 (H1N1)-like virus;
- an A/Wisconsin/67/2005 (H3N2)-like virus (A/Wisconsin/67/2005 and A/Hiroshima/52/2005 strains);
- a B/Malaysia/2506/2004-like virus from B/Malaysia/2506/2004 and B/Ohio/1/2005 strains which are of B/Victoria/2/87 lineage.

Flu Season 2007-2008

The composition of influenza virus vaccines for use in the 2007–2008 Northern Hemisphere influenza season recommended by the World Health Organisation on 14 February 2007 was:

- an A/Solomon Islands/3/2006 (H1N1)-like virus;
- an A/Wisconsin/67/2005 (H3N2)-like virus (A/Wisconsin/67/2005 (H3N2) and A/Hiroshima/52/2005 were used at the time);
- a B/Malaysia/2506/2004-like virus

"A/H3N2 has become the predominant flu subtype in the United States, and the record over the past 25 years shows that seasons dominated by H3N2 tend to be worse than those dominated by type A/H1N1 or type B." Many H3N2 viruses making people ill in this 2007-2008 flu season differ from the strains in the vaccine and may not be well covered by the vaccine strains. "The CDC has analysed 250 viruses this season to determine how well they match up with the vaccine, the report says. Of 65 H3N2 isolates, 53 (81%) were

> characterised as A/Brisbane/10/2007-like, a variant that has evolved [notably] from the H3N2 strain in the vaccine—A/Wisconsin/67/2005."

Outbreak of Swine in Philippine 2007

On August 20, 2007 Department of Agriculture officers investigated the outbreak (epizootic) of swine flu in Nueva Ecija and Central Luzon, Philippines. The mortality rate is less than 10 per cent for swine flu, unless there are complications like hog cholera. On July 27, 2007, the Philippine National Meat Inspection Service (NMIS) raised a hog cholera *"red alert"* warning over Metro Manila and 5 regions of Luzon after the disease spread to backyard pig farms in Bulacan and Pampanga, even if these tested negative for the swine flu virus.

Various Kinds of Disease

Of the three genera of influenza viruses that cause human flu, two also cause influenza in pigs, with Influenzavirus A being common in pigs and Influenzavirus C being rare. Influenzavirus B has not been reported in pigs. Within Influenzavirus A and Influenzavirus C, the strains found in pigs and humans are largely distinct, although due to reassortment there have been transfers of genes among strains crossing swine, avian, and human species boundaries.

Surveillance

Although there is no formal national surveillance system in the United States to determine what viruses are circulating in pigs, there is an informal surveillance network in the United States that is part of a world surveillance network.

Veterinary medical pathologist, Tracey McNamara, set up a national disease surveillance system in zoos because the zoos do active disease surveillance and many of the exotic animals housed there have broad susceptibilities. Many species fall below the radar of any federal agencies (including dogs, cats, pet prairie dogs, zoo animals, and urban wildlife), even though they may be important in the early detection of human disease outbreaks.

Transmission of the Disease

Transmission between Pigs

Influenza is quite common in pigs, with about half of breeding pigs having been exposed to the virus in the US. Antibodies to the virus are also common in pigs in other countries.

The main route of transmission is through direct contact between infected and uninfected animals. These close contacts are particularly common during animal transport. Intensive farming may also increase the risk of transmission, as the pigs are raised in very close proximity to each other. The direct transfer of the virus probably occurs either by pigs touching noses, or through dried mucus. Airborne transmission through the aerosols produced by pigs coughing or sneezing are also an important means of infection. The virus usually spreads quickly through a herd, infecting all the pigs within just a few days. Transmission may also occur through wild animals, such as wild boar, which can spread the disease between farms.

Transmission to Humans

People who work with poultry and swine, especially people with intense exposures, are at increased risk of zoonotic infection with influenza virus endemic in these animals, and constitute a population of human hosts in which zoonosis and reassortment can co-occur. Vaccination of these workers against influenza and surveillance for new influenza strains among this population may therefore be an important public health measure. Transmission of influenza from swine to humans who work with swine was documented in a small surveillance study performed in 2004 at the University of Iowa. This study among others forms the basis of a recommendation that people whose jobs involve handling poultry and swine be the focus of increased public health surveillance. Other professions at particular risk of infection are veterinarians and meat processing workers, although the risk of infection for both of these groups is lower than that of farm workers.

Interaction with Avian H5N1 in Pigs

Pigs are unusual as they can be infected with influenza strains that usually infect three different species: pigs, birds and humans. This makes pigs a host where influenza viruses might exchange genes, producing new and dangerous strains. H3N2 evolved from H2N2 by antigenic shift. In August 2004, researchers in China found H5N1 in pigs.

These H5N1 infections may be quite common: in a survey of 10 apparently healthy pigs housed near poultry farms in West Java, where avian flu had broken out, five of the pig samples contained the H5N1 virus. The Indonesian government has since found similar results in the same region. Additional tests of 150 pigs outside the area were negative.

Prevention of the Disease

Prevention of swine influenza has three components: prevention in swine, prevention of transmission to humans, and prevention of its spread among humans.

Prevention in Swine

Methods of preventing the spread of influenza among swine include facility management, herd management, and vaccination. Because much of the illness and death associated with swine flu involves secondary infection by other pathogens, control strategies that rely on vaccination may be insufficient.

Control of swine influenza by vaccination has become more difficult in recent decades, as the evolution of the virus has resulted in inconsistent responses to traditional vaccines. Standard commercial swine flu vaccines are effective in controlling the infection when the virus strains match enough to have significant cross-protection, and custom (autogenous) vaccines made from the specific viruses isolated are created and used in the more difficult cases. Present vaccination strategies for SIV control and prevention in swine farms typically include the use of one of several bivalent SIV vaccines commercially available in the United States. Of the 97 recent H3N2 isolates examined, only 41 isolates had strong serologic cross-reactions with antiserum to three commercial

SIV vaccines. Since the protective ability of influenza vaccines depends primarily on the closeness of the match between the vaccine virus and the epidemic virus, the presence of non-reactive H3N2 SIV variants suggests that current commercial vaccines might not effectively protect pigs from infection with a majority of H3N2 viruses. The United States Department of Agriculture researchers say that while pig vaccination keeps pigs from getting sick, it does not block infection or shedding of the virus.

Facility management includes using disinfectants and ambient temperature to control virus in the environment. The virus is unlikely to survive outside living cells for more than two weeks, except in cold (but above freezing) conditions, and it is readily inactivated by disinfectants. Herd management includes not adding pigs carrying influenza to herds that have not been exposed to the virus. The virus survives in healthy carrier pigs for up to 3 months and can be recovered from them between outbreaks. Carrier pigs are usually responsible for the introduction of SIV into previously uninfected herds and countries, so new animals should be quarantined. After an outbreak, as immunity in exposed pigs wanes, new outbreaks of the same strain can occur.

Prevention in Humans

Prevention of Pig to Human Transmission: The transmission from swine to human is believed to occur mainly in swine farms where farmers are in close contact with live pigs. Although strains of swine influenza are usually not able to infect humans this may occasionally happen, so farmers and veterinarians are encouraged to use a face mask when dealing with infected animals. The use of vaccines on swine to prevent their infection is a major method of limiting swine to human transmission. Risk factors that may contribute to swine-to-human transmission include smoking and not wearing gloves when working with sick animals.

Prevention of Human to Human Transmission: Influenza spreads between humans through coughing or sneezing and people touching something with the virus on it and then touching their own nose or mouth. Swine flu cannot be spread by pork products, since the virus is not transmitted through food. The swine flu in humans is most contagious during the first five days of the illness although some people, most commonly children, can remain contagious for up to ten days. Diagnosis can be made by sending a specimen, collected during the first five days for analysis.

Recommendations to prevent spread of the virus among humans include using standard infection control against influenza. This includes frequent washing of hands with soap and water or with alcohol-based hand sanitisers, especially after being out in public. Chance of transmission is also reduced by disinfecting household surfaces, which can be done effectively with a diluted chlorine bleach solution. Although the current trivalent influenza vaccine is unlikely to provide protection against the new 2009 H1N1 strain, vaccines against the new strain are being developed and could be ready as early as June 2009.

Experts agree that hand-washing can help prevent viral infections, including ordinary influenza and the swine flu virus. Influenza can spread in coughs or sneezes, but an increasing body of evidence shows small droplets containing the virus can linger on tabletops, telephones and other surfaces and be transferred via the fingers to the mouth, nose or eyes. Alcohol-based gel or foam hand sanitisers work well to destroy viruses and bacteria. Anyone with flu-like symptoms such as a sudden fever, cough or muscle aches should stay away from work or public transportation and should contact a doctor for advice.

Social distancing is another tactic. It means staying away from other people who might be infected and can include avoiding large gatherings, spreading out a little at work, or perhaps staying home and lying low if an infection is spreading in a community. Public health and other responsible authorities have action plans which may request or require social distancing actions depending on the severity of the outbreak.

Treatment of the Disease

In Swine

As swine influenza is rarely fatal to pigs, little treatment beyond rest and supportive care is required. Instead veterinary efforts are focused on preventing the spread of the virus throughout the farm, or to other farms. Vaccination and animal management techniques are most important in these efforts. Antibiotics are also used to treat this disease, which although they have no effect against the influenza virus, do help prevent bacterial pneumonia and other secondary infections in influenza-weakened herds.

In Humans

If a person becomes sick with swine flu, antiviral drugs can make the illness milder and make the patient feel better faster. They may also prevent serious flu complications. For treatment, antiviral drugs work best if started soon after getting sick (within 2 days of symptoms). Beside antivirals, palliative care, at home or in hospital, focuses on controlling fevers and maintaining fluid balance. The US Centres for Disease Control and Prevention recommends the use of Tamiflu (oseltamivir) or Relenza (zanamivir) for the treatment and/or prevention of infection with swine influenza viruses, however, the majority of people infected with the virus make a full recovery without requiring medical attention or antiviral drugs. The virus isolates in the 2009 outbreak have been found resistant to amantadine and rimantadine.

In the US, on April 27, 2009, the FDA issued Emergency Use Authorisations to make available Relenza and Tamiflu antiviral drugs to treat the swine influenza virus in cases for which they are currently unapproved. The agency issued these EUAs to allow treatment of patients younger than the current approval allows and to allow the widespread distribution of the drugs, including by non-licensed volunteers.

Orthomyxoviridae

The *Orthomyxoviridae* (*orthos*, Greek for "straight"; *myxa*, Greek for "mucus") are a family of RNA viruses that includes five genera: Influenzavirus A, Influenzavirus B, Influenzavirus

C, Isavirus and Thogotovirus. The first three genera contain viruses that cause influenza in vertebrates, including birds, humans, and other mammals. Isaviruses infect salmon; thogotoviruses infect vertebrates and invertebrates, such as mosquitoes and sea lice.

The three genera of Influenzavirus, which are identified by antigenic differences in their nucleoprotein and matrix protein infect vertebrates as follows:

- Influenzavirus A cause of all flu pandemics and infect humans, other mammals and birds
- Influenzavirus B infect humans and seals
- Influenzavirus C infect humans and pigs

Classification: In a phylogenetic-based taxonomy the "RNA viruses" includes the "negative-sense ssRNA viruses" which includes the Order "*Mononegavirales*", and the Family "*Orthomyxoviridae*" (among others). The species and serotypes of *Orthomyxoviridae* are shown in the following table.

Orthomyxoviridae Genera, Species, and Serotypes

Genus	*Species (indicates type species)*	*Serotypes or Subtypes*	*Hosts*
Influenzavirus A	Influenza A virus	H1N1, H1N2, H2N2, H3N1, H3N2, H3N8, H5N1, H5N2, H5N3, H5N8, H5N9, H7N1, H7N2, H7N3, H7N4, H7N7, H9N2, H10N7	Human, pig, bird, horse
Influenzavirus B	Influenza B virus		Human, seal
Influenzavirus C	Influenza C virus		Human, pig
Isavirus	Infectious salmon anaemia virus		Atlantic salmon
Thogotovirus	Thogoto virus Dhori virus	Batken virus, Dhori virus	Tick, mosquito, mammal (including human)

2

Influenza, the Disease

Etymology

Influenza, commonly referred to as the flu, is an infectious disease caused by RNA viruses of the family Orthomyxoviridae (the influenza viruses), that affects birds and mammals. The name *influenza* comes from the Italian *influenza*, meaning "influence" (Latin: *influentia*). The most common symptoms of the disease are chills, fever, sore throat, muscle pains, severe headache, coughing, weakness and general discomfort. Fever and coughs are the most frequent symptoms. In more serious cases, influenza causes pneumonia, which can be fatal, particularly for the young and the elderly. Although it is often confused with other influenza-like illnesses, especially the common cold, influenza is a much more severe disease than the common cold and is caused by a different type of virus. Influenza may produce nausea and vomiting, particularly in children, but these symptoms are more common in the unrelated gastroenteritis, which is sometimes called "stomach flu" or "24-hour flu".

Typically, influenza is transmitted through the air by coughs or sneezes, creating aerosols containing the virus. Influenza can also be transmitted by bird droppings, saliva, nasal secretions, feces and blood. Infection can also occur through contact with these body fluids or through contact with contaminated surfaces. Airborne aerosols have been thought to cause most infections, although which means of transmission is most important is not absolutely clear. Influenza viruses can be inactivated by sunlight, disinfectants and detergents. As the virus can be inactivated by soap, frequent hand washing reduces the risk of infection.

Influenza spreads around the world in seasonal epidemics, resulting in the deaths of hundreds of thousands annually — millions in pandemic years. Three influenza pandemics occurred in the 20th century and killed tens of millions of people, with each of these pandemics being caused by the appearance of a new strain of the virus in humans. Often, these new strains appear when an existing flu virus spreads to humans from other animal species, or when an existing human strain picks up new genes from an a virus that usually infects birds or pigs. An avian strain named H5N1 raised the concern of a new influenza pandemic, after it emerged in Asia in the 1990s, but it has not evolved to a form that spreads easily between people. In April 2009 a novel flu strain evolved that combined genes from human, pig, and bird flu, initially dubbed "swine flu", emerged in Mexico, the United States, and several other nations. By late-April, the new strain was suspected of having killed over 150 in Mexico, and prompted concern that a new pandemic is imminent. However, confirmed cases were lower, with only 10 deaths by the end of April, 9 in Mexico and only 1 in the both the US and Canada.

Vaccinations against influenza are usually given to people in developed countries and to farmed poultry. The most common human vaccine is the trivalent influenza vaccine (TIV) that contains purified and inactivated material from three viral strains. Typically, this vaccine includes material from two influenza A virus subtypes and one influenza B virus strain. The TIV carries no risk of transmitting the disease, and it has very low reactivity. A vaccine formulated for one year may be ineffective in the following year, since the influenza virus evolves rapidly, and new strains quickly replace the older ones. Antiviral drugs can be used to treat influenza, with neuraminidase inhibitors being particularly effective.

Influenzavirus

The word *Influenza* comes from the Italian language and refers to the cause of the disease; initially, this ascribed illness to unfavourable astrological influences. Changes in medical thought led to its modification to *influenza del freddo*, meaning "influence of the cold". The word *influenza* was first used in English in 1743 when it was adopted, with an anglicised pronunciation, during an outbreak of the disease in Europe. Archaic terms for influenza include *epidemic catarrh, grippe* (from the French), *sweating sickness*, and *Spanish fever* (particularly for the 1918 pandemic strain).

History

The symptoms of human influenza were clearly described by Hippocrates roughly 2,400 years ago. Since then, the virus has caused numerous pandemics. Historical data on influenza are difficult to interpret, because the symptoms can be similar to those of other diseases, such as diphtheria, pneumonic plague, typhoid fever, dengue, or typhus. The first convincing record of an influenza pandemic was of an outbreak in 1580, which began in Russia and spread to Europe via Africa. In Rome, over 8,000 people were killed, and several Spanish cities were almost wiped out. Pandemics continued sporadically throughout the 17th and 18th centuries, with the pandemic of 1830–1833 being particularly widespread; it infected approximately a quarter of the people exposed.

The most famous and lethal outbreak was the so-called Spanish flu pandemic (type A influenza, H1N1 subtype), which lasted from 1918 to 1919. It is not known exactly how many it killed, but estimates range from 20 to 100 million people. This pandemic has been described as "the greatest medical holocaust in history" and may have killed as many people as the Black Death.

The Spanish flu pandemic was truly global, spreading even to the Arctic and remote Pacific islands. The unusually severe disease killed between 2 and 20 per cent of those infected, as opposed to the more usual flu epidemic mortality rate of 0.1 per cent. Another unusual feature of this pandemic was that it mostly killed young adults, with 99 per cent of pandemic influenza deaths occurring in people under 65, and more than half in young adults 20 to 40 years old. This is unusual since influenza is normally most deadly to the very young (under age 2) and the very old (over age 70). The total mortality of the 1918–1919 pandemic is not known, but it is estimated that 2.5 per cent to 5 per cent of the world's population was killed. As many as 25 million may have been killed in the first 25 weeks; in contrast, HIV/AIDS has killed 25 million in its first 25 years.

Later flu pandemics were not so devastating. They included the 1957 Asian Flu (type A, H2N2 strain) and the 1968 Hong Kong Flu (type A, H3N2 strain), but even these smaller outbreaks killed millions of people. In later pandemics antibiotics were available to control secondary infections and this may have helped reduce mortality compared to the Spanish Flu of 1918.

Known Flu Pandemics

Name of pandemic	*Date*	*Deaths*	*Subtype involved*	*Pandemic Severity Index*
Asiatic (Russian) Flu	1889–1890	1 million	possibly H2N2	?
Spanish Flu	1918–1920	20 to 100 million	H1N1	5
Asian Flu	1957–1958	1 to 1.5 million	H2N2	2
Hong Kong Flu	1968–1969	0.75 to 1 million	H3N2	2
2009 Flu Pandemic	2009-present	?	H1N1	?

The first influenza virus to be isolated was from poultry, when in 1901 the agent causing a disease called "fowl plague" was shown to be able to pass through a Chamberland filter, which have pores that are too small for bacteria to pass through. The aetiological cause of influenza, the Orthomyxoviridae family of viruses, was first discovered in pigs by Richard

Shope in 1931. This discovery was shortly followed by the isolation of the virus from humans by a group headed by Patrick Laidlaw at the Medical Research Council of the United Kingdom in 1933. However, it was not until Wendell Stanley first crystallised tobacco mosaic virus in 1935 that the non-cellular nature of viruses was appreciated.

The first significant step towards preventing influenza was the development in 1944 of a killed-virus vaccine for influenza by Thomas Francis, Jr.. This built on work by Australian Frank Macfarlane Burnet, who showed that the virus lost virulence when it was cultured in fertilized hen's eggs. Application of this observation by Francis allowed his group of researchers at the University of Michigan to develop the first influenza vaccine, with support from the US Army. The Army was deeply involved in this research due to its experience of influenza in World War I, when thousands of troops were killed by the virus in a matter of months. In comparison to vaccines, the development of anti-influenza drugs has been slower, with amantadine being licensed in 1966 and, almost thirty years later, the next class of drugs (the neuraminidase inhibitors) being developed.

Although there were scares in the US state of New Jersey in 1976 (with a strain of Swine Flu), worldwide in 1977 (with the Russian Flu), and in Hong Kong and other Asian countries in 1997 (with H5N1 avian influenza), there have been no major pandemics since the 1968 Hong Kong Flu. Immunity to previous pandemic influenza strains and vaccination may have limited the spread of the virus and may have helped prevent further pandemics.

Microbiology

Types of Influenza Virus: In virus classification the influenza virus is an RNA virus of the family Orthomyxoviridae, which comprises five genera:

- Influenzavirus A
- Influenzavirus B

- Influenzavirus C
- Isavirus
- Thogotovirus

These viruses are only distantly related to the human parainfluenza viruses, which are RNA viruses belonging to the paramyxovirus family that are a common cause of respiratory infections in children such as croup, but can also cause a disease similar to influenza in adults.

Influenzavirus A

This genus has one species, influenza A virus. Wild aquatic birds are the natural hosts for a large variety of influenza A. Occasionally, viruses are transmitted to other species and may then cause devastating outbreaks in domestic poultry or give rise to human influenza pandemics. The type A viruses are the most virulent human pathogens among the three influenza types and cause the most severe disease. The influenza A virus can be subdivided into different serotypes based on the antibody response to these viruses. The serotypes that have been confirmed in humans, ordered by the number of known human pandemic deaths, are:

- H1N1, which caused Spanish flu in 1918, and Swine flu in 2009
- H2N2, which caused Asian Flu in 1957
- H3N2, which caused Hong Kong Flu in 1968
- H5N1, a pandemic threat in the 2007–08 flu season
- H7N7, which has unusual zoonotic potential
- H1N2, endemic in humans and pigs
- H9N2
- H7N2
- H7N3
- H10N7

In 2009, a recombinant influenza virus derived in part from H1N1 was first detected in Mexico and the United States.

Influenzavirus B

This genus has one species, influenza B virus. Influenza B almost exclusively infects humans and is less common than influenza A. The only other animals known to be susceptible to influenza B infection are the seal and the ferret. This type of influenza mutates at a rate 2–3 times lower than type A and consequently is less genetically diverse, with only one influenza B serotype. As a result of this lack of antigenic diversity, a degree of immunity to influenza B is usually acquired at an early age. However, influenza B mutates enough that lasting immunity is not possible. This reduced rate of antigenic change, combined with its limited host range (inhibiting cross species antigenic shift), ensures that pandemics of influenza B do not occur.

Influenzavirus C

This genus has one species, influenza C virus, which infects humans, dogs and pigs, sometimes causing both severe illness and local epidemics. However, influenza C is less common than the other types and usually seems to cause mild disease in children.

Structure, Properties and Subtype Nomenclature

Influenzaviruses A, B and C are very similar in overall structure. The virus particle is 80-120 nanometres in diameter and usually roughly spherical, although filamentous forms can occur. These filamentous forms are more common in influenza C, which can form cordlike structures up to 500 micrometres long on the surfaces of infected cells. However, despite these varied shapes, the viral particles of all influenza viruses are similar in composition. These are made of a viral envelope containing two main types of glycoproteins, wrapped around a central core. The central core contains the viral RNA genome and other viral proteins that package and protect this RNA. Unusually for a virus, its genome is not a single piece of nucleic acid; instead, it contains seven or eight pieces of segmented negative-sense RNA, each piece of RNA contains either one or two genes. For example, the influenza A genome contains 11 genes on eight pieces of RNA, encoding for 11 proteins: hemagglutinin (HA), neuraminidase (NA), nucleoprotein (NP), M1, M2, NS1, NS2(NEP), PA, PB1, PB1-F2 and PB2.

Hemagglutinin (HA) and neuraminidase (NA) are the two large glycoproteins on the outside of the viral particles. HA is a lectin that mediates binding of the virus to target cells and entry of the viral genome into the target cell, while NA is involved in the release of progeny virus from infected cells, by cleaving sugars that bind the mature viral particles. Thus, these proteins are targets for antiviral drugs. Furthermore, they are antigens to which antibodies can be raised. Influenza A viruses are classified into subtypes based on antibody responses to HA and NA. These different types of HA and NA form the basis of the *H* and *N* distinctions in, for example, *H5N1*. There are 16 H and 9 N subtypes known, but only H 1, 2 and 3, and N 1 and 2 are commonly found in humans.

Replication: Viruses can only replicate in living cells. Influenza infection and replication is a multi-step process: firstly the virus has to bind to and enter the cell, then deliver its genome to a site where it can produce new copies of viral proteins and RNA, assemble these components into new viral particles and finally exit the host cell.

Influenza viruses bind through hemagglutinin onto sialic acid sugars on the surfaces of epithelial cells; typically in the nose, throat and lungs of mammals and intestines of birds. After the hemagglutinin is cleaved by a protease, the cell imports the virus by endocytosis.

Once inside the cell, the acidic conditions in the endosome cause two events to happen: first part of the hemagglutinin protein fuses the viral envelope with the vacuole's membrane, then the M2 ion channel allows protons to move through the viral envelope and acidify the core of the virus, which causes the core to dissemble and release the viral RNA and core proteins. The viral RNA (vRNA) molecules, accessory proteins and RNA-dependent RNA polymerase are then released into the cytoplasm. The M2 ion channel is blocked by amantadine drugs, preventing infection.

These core proteins and vRNA form a complex that is transported into the cell nucleus, where the RNA-dependent RNA polymerase begins transcribing complementary positive-sense vRNA. The vRNA is either exported into the cytoplasm and translated or remains in the nucleus. Newly synthesised viral proteins are either secreted through the Golgi apparatus onto the cell surface (in the case of neuraminidase and hemagglutinin) or transported back into the nucleus to bind vRNA and form new viral genome particles. Other viral proteins have multiple actions in the host cell, including degrading cellular mRNA and using the released nucleotides for vRNA synthesis and also inhibiting translation of host-cell mRNAs.

Negative-sense vRNAs that form the genomes of future viruses, RNA-dependent RNA polymerase, and other viral proteins are assembled into a virion. Hemagglutinin and neuraminidase molecules cluster into a bulge in the cell membrane. The vRNA and viral core proteins leave the nucleus and enter this membrane protrusion. The mature virus buds off from the cell in a sphere of host phospholipid membrane, acquiring hemagglutinin and neuraminidase with this membrane coat. As before, the viruses adhere to the cell through hemagglutinin; the mature viruses detach once their neuraminidase has cleaved sialic acid residues from the host cell. Drugs that inhibit neuraminidase, such as oseltamivir, therefore prevent the release of new infectious viruses and halt viral replication. After the release of new influenza viruses, the host cell dies.

Because of the absence of RNA proofreading enzymes, the RNA-dependent RNA polymerase that copies the viral genome makes an error roughly every 10 thousand nucleotides, which is the approximate length of the influenza vRNA. Hence, the majority of newly manufactured influenza viruses are mutants, this causes "antigenic drift", which is a slow change in the antigens on the viral surface over time. The separation of the genome into eight separate segments of vRNA allows mixing or reassortment of vRNAs if more than one type of influenza virus infects a single cell. The resulting rapid change in viral genetics produces antigenic shifts, which are sudden changes from one antigen to another. These sudden large changes allow the virus to infect new host species and quickly overcome protective immunity.

Transmission: People who contract influenza are most infective between the second and third days after infection and infectivity lasts for around ten days. Children are much more infectious than adults and shed virus from just before they develop symptoms until two weeks after infection. The transmission of influenza can be modelled mathematically, which helps predict how the virus will spread in a population.

Influenza can be spread in three main ways: by direct transmission when an infected person sneezes mucus into the eyes, nose or mouth of another person; through people inhaling the aerosols produced by infected people coughing, sneezing and spitting; and through hand-to-mouth transmission from either contaminated surfaces or direct personal contact, such as a handshake. The relative importance of these three modes of transmission is unclear, and they may all contribute to the spread of the virus. In the airborne route, the droplets that are small enough for people to inhale are 0.5 to 5 μm in diameter and inhaling just one droplet might be enough to cause an infection. Although a single sneeze releases up to 40,000 droplets, most of these droplets are quite large and will quickly settle out of the air. How long influenza survives in airborne droplets seems to be influenced by the levels of humidity and UV radiation: with low humidity and a lack of sunlight in winter probably aiding its survival.

As the influenza virus can persist outside of the body, it can also be transmitted by contaminated surfaces such as banknotes, doorknobs, light switches and other household items. The length of time the virus will persist on a surface varies, with the virus surviving for one to two days on hard, non-porous surfaces such as plastic or metal, for about fifteen minutes from dry paper tissues, and only five minutes on skin. However, if the virus is present in mucus, this can protect it for longer periods. Avian influenza viruses can survive indefinitely when frozen. They are inactivated by heating to 56°C (133°F) for a minimum of 60 minutes, as well as by acids (at pH <2).

Symptoms and Diagnosis

Symptoms of influenza can start quite suddenly one to two days after infection. Usually the first symptoms are chills or a chilly sensation, but fever is also common early in the infection, with body temperatures ranging from 38-39°C (approximately 100-103°F). Many people are so ill that they are confined to bed for several days, with aches and pains throughout their bodies, which are worse in their backs and legs. Symptoms of influenza may include:

- Body aches, especially joints and throat.
- Extreme coldness and fever.
- Fatigue.
- Headache.
- Irritated watering eyes.
- Reddened eyes, skin (especially face), mouth, throat and nose.
- Abdominal pain (in children with influenza B).

It can be difficult to distinguish between the common cold and influenza in the early stages of these infections, but a flu can be identified by a high fever with a sudden onset and extreme fatigue. Diarrhoea is not normally a symptom of influenza in adults, although it has been seen in some human cases of the H5N1 "bird flu" and can be a symptom in children. The symptoms most reliably seen in influenza are shown in the table.

Most Sensitive Symptoms for Diagnosing Influenza

Symptom	*Sensitivity*	*Specificity*
Fever	68-86%	25-73%
Cough	84-98%	7-29%
Nasal congestion	68-91%	19-41%

Notes to table:

- The ranges given represent different studies that were reviewed.
- Sensitivity is the proportion of people having influenza who exhibit the symptom.
- Specificity is the proportion of people not having influenza who do not exhibit the symptom.
- All three findings, especially fever, were less sensitive in patients over 60 years of age.

Since antiviral drugs are effective in treating influenza if given early, it can be important to identify cases early. Of the symptoms listed above, the combinations of fever with cough, sore throat and/or nasal conjestion can improve diagnostic accuracy. Two decision analysis studies suggest that *during local outbreaks* of influenza, the prevalence will be over 70 per cent, and thus patients with any of these combinations of symptoms may be treated with neuramidase inhibitors without testing. Even in the absence of a local outbreak, treatment may be justified in the elderly during the influenza season as long as the prevalence is over 15 per cent.

Laboratory Tests

The available laboratory tests for influenza continue to get better. The United States Centres for Disease Control and Prevention (CDC) maintains an up-to-date summary of available laboratory tests. According to the CDC, rapid diagnostic tests have a sensitivity of 70-75 per cent and specificity of 90-95 per cent when compared with viral culture. These tests may be especially useful during the influenza season (prevalence=25%) but in the absence of a local outbreak, or peri-influenza season (prevalence=10%).

Prognosis

Influenza's effects are much more severe and last longer than those of the common cold. Most people will recover completely in about one to two weeks, but others will develop life-threatening complications (such as pneumonia). Influenza, however, can be deadly, especially for the weak, old, or chronically ill. People with a weak immune system, such as people infected with HIV or transplant patients (whose immune systems are medically suppressed to prevent transplant organ rejection), suffer from particularly severe disease. Other high-risk groups include pregnant women and young children.

The flu can worsen chronic health problems. People with emphysema, chronic bronchitis or asthma may experience shortness of breath while they have the flu, and influenza may cause worsening of coronary heart disease or congestive heart failure. Smoking is another risk factor associated with more serious disease and increased mortality from influenza.

According to the World Health Organisation: "Every winter, tens of millions of people get the flu. Most are only ill and out of work for a week, yet the elderly are at a higher risk of death from the illness. We know the worldwide death toll exceeds a few hundred thousand people a year, but even in developed countries the numbers are uncertain, because medical authorities don't usually verify who actually died of influenza and who died of a flu-like illness." Even healthy people can be affected, and serious problems from influenza can happen at any age. People over 50 years old, very young children and people of any age with chronic medical conditions are more likely to get complications from influenza, such as pneumonia, bronchitis, sinus, and ear infections.

In some cases, an autoimmune response to an influenza infection may contribute to the development of Guillain-Barré syndrome. However, as many other infections can increase the risk of this disease, influenza may only be an important cause during epidemics. This syndrome can also be a rare side-effect of influenza vaccines, with an incidence of about one case per million vaccinations.

Pathophysiology

The mechanisms by which influenza infection causes symptoms in humans have been studied intensively. Consequently, knowing which genes are carried by a particular strain can help predict how well it will infect humans and how severe this infection will be (that is, predict the strain's pathophysiology). For instance, part of the process that allows influenza viruses to invade cells is the cleavage of the viral hemagglutinin protein by any one of several human proteases. In mild and avirulent viruses, the structure of the hemagglutinin means that it can only be cleaved by proteases found in the throat and lungs, so these viruses cannot infect other tissues. However, in highly virulent strains, such as H5N1, the hemagglutinin can be cleaved by a wide variety of proteases, allowing the virus to spread throughout the body. The H1N1 virus responsible for the 2009 swine flu outbreak appears to have a cleavage site that would limit its spread and reduce its virulence.

The viral hemagglutinin protein is also responsible for determining where in the respiratory tract a particular strain of influenza will bind. Strains that are easily transmitted between people, but which usually cause mild disease, have hemagglutinin proteins that bind to receptors in the upper part of the respiratory tract, such as in the nose, throat and mouth. In contrast, virulent strains such as H5N1 bind to receptors that are mostly found deep in the lungs. This difference in the site of infection may explain why the H5N1 strain causes severe viral pneumonia in the lungs, but is not easily transmitted between people through coughing and sneezing.

Common symptoms of the flu such as fever, headaches, and fatigue come from the huge amounts of proinflammatory cytokines and chemokines (such as interferon or tumour necrosis factor) produced from influenza-infected cells. In contrast to the rhinovirus that causes the common cold, influenza does cause tissue damage, so symptoms are not entirely due to the inflammatory response. This massive immune response might produce a life-threatening cytokine storm. This effect has been proposed to be the cause of the unusual lethality of both the H5N1 avian influenza, and the 1918 pandemic strain. However, another possibility is that these large amounts of cytokines are just a result of the massive levels of viral replication produced by these strains, and the immune response does not itself contribute to the disease.

Epidemiology

Seasonal Variations: Influenza reaches peak prevalence in winter, and because the Northern and Southern Hemispheres have winter at different times of the year, there are actually two different flu seasons each year. This is why the World Health Organisation (assisted by the National Influenza Centres) makes recommendations for two different vaccine formulations every year; one for the Northern, and one for the Southern Hemisphere.

It is not clear why outbreaks of the flu occur seasonally rather than uniformly throughout the year. One possible explanation is that, because people are indoors more often during the winter, they are in close contact more often, and this promotes transmission from person to person. Another is that cold temperatures lead to drier air, which may dehydrate mucus, preventing the body from effectively expelling virus particles. The virus may also survive longer on exposed surfaces (doorknobs, countertops, etc.) in colder temperatures. Increased travel due to the Northern Hemisphere winter holiday season may also play a role. A contributing factor is that aerosol transmission of the virus is highest in cold environments (less than 5 °C) with low humidity. However, seasonal changes in infection rates also occur in tropical regions, and these peaks of infection are seen mainly during the rainy season. Seasonal changes in contact rates from school terms, which are a major factor in other childhood diseases such as measles and pertussis, may also play a role in the flu. A combination of these small seasonal effects may be amplified by dynamical resonance with the endogenous disease cycles. H5N1 exhibits seasonality in both humans and birds.

An alternative hypothesis to explain seasonality in influenza infections is an effect of vitamin D levels on immunity to the virus. This idea was first proposed by Robert Edgar Hope-Simpson in 1965. He proposed that the cause of influenza epidemics during winter may be connected to seasonal fluctuations of vitamin D, which is produced in the skin under the influence of solar (or artificial) UV radiation. This could explain why influenza occurs mostly in winter and during the tropical rainy season, when people stay indoors, away from the sun, and their vitamin D levels fall.

3

Types of the Disease

Various Influenza

There are three genera of influenza virus: Influenzavirus A, Influenzavirus B and Influenzavirus C. Each genus includes only one species, or type: Influenza A virus, Influenza B virus, and Influenza C virus, respectively. Influenza A and C infect multiple species, while influenza B almost exclusively infects humans.

Influenza A

Influenza A viruses are further classified, based on the viral surface proteins hemagglutinin (HA or H) and neuraminidase (NA or N). Sixteen H subtypes (or serotypes) and nine N subtypes of influenza A virus have been identified.

Further variation exists; thus, specific influenza strain isolates are identified by a standard nomenclature specifying virus type, geographical location where first isolated, sequential number of isolation, year of isolation, and HA and NA subtype.

Examples of the nomenclature are:

1. A/Moscow/10/99 (H3N2)
2. B/Hong Kong/330/2001

The type A viruses are the most virulent human pathogens among the three influenza types and causes the most severe disease. The serotypes that have been confirmed in humans, ordered by the number of known human pandemic deaths, are:

- H1N1 caused "Spanish Flu".
- H2N2 caused "Asian Flu".
- H3N2 caused "Hong Kong Flu".
- H5N1 was a pandemic threat in 2006-7 flu season.
- H7N7 has unusual zoonotic potential.
- H1N2 is endemic in humans and pigs.
- H9N2, H7N2, H7N3, H10N7.

Flu Pandemics

Name	*Year*	*Deaths (millions)*	*Subtype involved*
Asiatic (Russian) Flu	1889-90	1	possibly H2N2
Spanish Flu	1918-20	40	H1N1
Asian Flu	1957-58	1-1.5	H2N2
Hong Kong Flu	1968-69	0.75	H3N2

Influenza B

Influenza B virus is almost exclusively a human pathogen, and is less common than influenza A. The only other animal known to be susceptible to influenza B infection is the seal. This type of influenza mutates at a rate 2-3 times lower than type A and consequently is less genetically diverse, with only one influenza B serotype. As a result of this lack of antigenic diversity, a degree of immunity to influenza B is usually acquired at an early age. However, influenza B mutates enough that lasting immunity is not possible. This reduced rate of antigenic change, combined with its limited host range (inhibiting cross species antigenic shift), ensures that pandemics of influenza B do not occur.

Influenza C

The influenza C virus infects humans and pigs, and can cause severe illness and local epidemics. However, influenza

C is less common than the other types and usually seems to cause mild disease in children.

Virology

Morphology: The virion is pleomorphic, the envelope can occur in spherical and filamentous forms. In general the virus's morphology is spherical with particles 50 to 120 nm in diameter, or filamentous virions 20 nm in diameter and 200 to 300 (-3000) nm long. There are some 500 distinct spike-like surface projections of the envelope each projecting 10 to 14 nm from the surface with some types [i.e. hemagglutinin esterase (HEF)] densely dispersed over the surface, and with others [i.e. hemagglutinin (HA)] spaced widely apart.

The major glycoprotein (HA) is interposed irregularly by clusters of neuraminidase (NA), with a ratio of HA to NA of about 4-5 to 1.

Lipoprotein membranes enclose the nucleocapsids; nucleoproteins of different size classes with a loop at each end; the arrangement within the virion is uncertain. The nucleocapsids are filamentous and fall in the range of 50 to 130 nm long and 9 to 15 nm in diameter. They have a helical symmetry.

Genome: Viruses of this family contain 7 to 8 segments of linear negative-sense single stranded RNA.

The total genome length is 12000-15000 nucleotides (nt). The largest segment 2300-2500 nt; of second largest 2300-2500 nt; of third 2200-2300 nt; of fourth 1700-1800 nt; of fifth 1500-1600 nt; of sixth 1400-1500 nt; of seventh 1000-1100 nt; of eighth 800-900 nt. Genome sequence has terminal repeated sequences; repeated at both ends. Terminal repeats at the 5'-end 12-13 nucleotides long. Nucleotide sequences of 3'-terminus identical; the same in genera of same family; most on RNA (segments), or on all RNA species. Terminal repeats at the 3'-end 9-11 nucleotides long. Encapsidated nucleic acid is solely genomic. Each virion may contain defective interfering copies.

Structure: For an in-depth example.

The following applies for Influenza A viruses, although other influenza strains are very similar in structure:

The influenza A virus particle or *virion* is 80-120 nm in diameter and usually roughly spherical, although filamentous forms can occur. Unusually for a virus, the influenza A genome is not a single piece of nucleic acid; instead, it contains eight pieces of segmented negative-sense RNA (13.5 kilobases total), which encode 11 proteins (HA, NA, NP, M1, M2, NS1, NEP, PA, PB1, PB1-F2, PB2). The best-characterised of these viral proteins are hemagglutinin and neuraminidase, two large glycoproteins found on the outside of the viral particles. Neuraminidase is an enzyme involved in the release of progeny virus from infected cells, by cleaving sugars that bind the mature viral particles. By contrast, hemagglutinin is a lectin that mediates binding of the virus to target cells and entry of the viral genome into the target cell. The hemagglutinin (H) and neuraminidase (N) proteins are targets for antiviral drugs. These proteins are also recognised by antibodies, i.e. they are antigens. The responses of antibodies to these proteins are used to classify the different serotypes of influenza A viruses, hence the *H* and *N* in *H5N1*.

Life Cycle: Typically, influenza is transmitted from infected mammals through the air by coughs or sneezes, creating aerosols containing the virus, and from infected birds through their droppings. Influenza can also be transmitted by saliva, nasal secretions, feces and blood. Infections occur through contact with these bodily fluids or with contaminated surfaces. Flu viruses can remain infectious for about one week at human body temperature, over 30 days at 0 °C (32 °F), and indefinitely at very low temperatures (such as lakes in northeast Siberia). They can be inactivated easily by disinfectants and detergents.

The viruses bind to a cell through interactions between its hemagglutinin glycoprotein and sialic acid sugars on the surfaces of epithelial cells in the lung and throat. The cell imports the virus by endocytosis. In the acidic endosome, part of the haemagglutinin protein fuses the viral envelope with the vacuole's membrane, releasing the viral RNA (vRNA) molecules, accessory proteins and RNA-dependent RNA polymerase into the cytoplasm. These proteins and vRNA form a complex that is transported into the cell nucleus, where the RNA-dependent RNA transcriptase begins transcribing complementary positive-sense vRNA. The vRNA is either exported into the cytoplasm and translated, or remains in the nucleus. Newly-synthesised viral proteins are either secreted through the Golgi apparatus onto the cell surface (in the case of neuraminidase and hemagglutinin) or transported back into the nucleus to bind vRNA and form new viral genome particles. Other viral proteins have multiple actions in the host cell, including degrading cellular mRNA and using the released nucleotides for vRNA synthesis and also inhibiting translation of host-cell mRNAs.

Negative-sense vRNAs that form the genomes of future viruses, RNA-dependent RNA transcriptase, and other viral proteins are assembled into a virion. Hemagglutinin and neuraminidase molecules cluster into a bulge in the cell membrane. The vRNA and viral core proteins leave the nucleus and enter this membrane protrusion. The mature virus buds off from the cell in a sphere of host phospholipid membrane, acquiring hemagglutinin and neuraminidase with this membrane coat. As before, the viruses adhere to the cell through hemagglutinin; the mature viruses detach once their neuraminidase has cleaved sialic acid residues from the host cell. After the release of new influenza virus, the host cell dies.

Since RNA proofreading enzymes are absent, the RNA-dependent RNA transcriptase makes a single nucleotide insertion error roughly every 10 thousand nucleotides, which is the approximate length of the influenza vRNA. Hence, nearly every newly-manufactured influenza virus will contain a mutation in its genome. The separation of the genome into eight separate segments of vRNA allows mixing (reassortment) of the genes if more than one variety of influenza virus has infected the same cell (superinfection). The resulting alteration in the genome segments packaged in to viral progeny confers new behaviour, sometimes the ability to infect new host species or to overcome protective immunity of host populations to its old genome (in which case it is called an antigenic shift).

Viability and Disinfection: Mammalian influenza virus tend to be labile, but can survive several hours in mucus. Avian influenza virus can survive for 100 days in distilled water at room temperature, and 200 days at 17 °C (63 °F). The avian virus is inactivated more quickly in manure, but can survive for up to 2 weeks in feces on cages. Avian influenza viruses can survive indefinitely when frozen. Influenza viruses are susceptible to bleach, 70 per cent ethanol, aldehydes, oxidising agents, and quaternary ammonium compounds. They are inactivated by heat of 133 °F (56 °C) for minimum of 60 minutes, as well as by low pH <2.

Influenzavirus A

Influenzavirus A is a genus of the Orthomyxoviridae family of viruses. Influenzavirus A includes only one species: *Influenza A virus* which causes influenza in birds and some mammals. Strains of all subtypes of influenza A virus have been isolated from wild birds, although disease is uncommon. Some isolates of influenza A virus cause severe disease both in domestic poultry and, rarely, in humans. Occasionally viruses are transmitted from wild aquatic birds to domestic poultry and this may cause an outbreak or give rise to human influenza pandemics.

Influenza A viruses are negative sense, single-stranded, segmented RNA viruses. There are several subtypes, labelled according to an H number (for the type of hemagglutinin) and an N number (for the type of neuraminidase). There are 16 different H antigens (H1 to H16) and nine different N antigens (N1 to N9). The newest H type (H16) was isolated from black-headed gulls caught in Sweden and the Netherlands in 1999 and reported in the literature in 2005.

Each virus subtype has mutated into a variety of strains with differing pathogenic profiles; some pathogenic to one species but not others, some pathogenic to multiple species.

Variants and Subtypes

Variants are identified and named according to the isolate that they are like and thus are presumed to share lineage (example Fujian flu virus like); according to their typical host (example Human flu virus); according to their subtype (example H3N2); and according to their deadliness (example LP, Low Pathogenic). So a flu from a virus similar to the isolate A/Fujian/411/2002(H3N2) is called Fujian flu, human flu, and H3N2 flu.

Variants are sometimes named according to the species (host) the strain is endemic in or adapted to. The main variants named using this convention are:

- Bird flu
- Human flu
- Swine flu
- Horse flu
- Dog flu
- Cat flu

Variants have also sometimes been named according to their deadliness in poultry, especially chickens:

- Low Pathogenic Avian Influenza (LPAI)
- Highly Pathogenic Avian Influenza (HPAI), also called: deadly flu or death flu

Most known strains are extinct strains. For example, the annual flu subtype H3N2 no longer contains the strain that caused the Hong Kong Flu.

Annual Flu

The annual flu (also called "seasonal flu" or "human flu") in the US "results in approximately 36,000 deaths and more than 200,000 hospitalisations each year. In addition to this human toll, influenza is annually responsible for a total cost of over $10 billion in the US" .

The annually updated trivalent influenza vaccine consists of hemagglutinin (HA) surface glycoprotein components from influenza H3N2, H1N1, and B influenza viruses.

The dominant strain in January 2006 is H3N2. Measured resistance to the standard antiviral drugs amantadine and rimantadine in H3N2 has increased from 1 per cent in 1994 to 12 per cent in 2003 to 91 per cent in 2005.

> "Contemporary human H3N2 influenza viruses are now endemic in pigs in southern China and can reassort with avian H5N1 viruses in this intermediate host."

Structure and Genetics

> "The physical structure of all influenza A viruses is similar. The virions or virus particles are enveloped and can be either spherical or filamentous in form. In clinical isolates that have undergone limited passages in eggs or tissue culture, there are more filamentous than spherical particles, whereas passaged laboratory strains consist mainly of spherical virions."

The Influenza A virus genome is contained on eight single (non-paired) RNA strands that code for eleven proteins (HA, NA, NP, M1, M2, NS1, NEP, PA, PB1, PB1-F2, PB2). The total genome size is 13,588 bases. The segmented nature of the genome allows for the exchange of entire genes between different viral strains during cellular cohabitation. The eight RNA segments are:

- HA encodes hemagglutinin (about 500 molecules of hemagglutinin are needed to make one virion) "The extent of infection into host organism is determined by HA. Influenza viruses bud from the apical surface of polarised epithelial cells (e.g. bronchial epithelial cells) into lumen of lungs and are therefore usually pneumotropic. The reason is that HA is cleaved by tryptase clara which is restricted to lungs. However,

HAs of H5 and H7 pantropic avian viruses subtypes can be cleaved by furin and subtilisin-type enzymes, allowing the virus to grow in other organs than lungs."

- NA encodes neuraminidase (about 100 molecules of neuraminidase are needed to make one virion).
- NP encodes nucleoprotein.
- M encodes two matrix proteins (the M1 and the M2) by using different reading frames from the same RNA segment (about 3000 matrix protein molecules are needed to make one virion).
- NS encodes two distinct non-structural proteins (NS1 and NEP) by using different reading frames from the same RNA segment.
- PA encodes an RNA polymerase.
- PB1 encodes an RNA polymerase and PB1-F2 protein (induces apoptosis) by using different reading frames from the same RNA segment.
- PB2 encodes an RNA polymerase.

The genome segments have common terminal sequences, and the ends of the RNA strands are partially complementary, allowing them to bond to each other by hydrogen bonds. After transcription from negative-sense to positive-sense RNA the +RNA strands get the cellular 5' cap added by cap snatching, which involves the viral protein NS1 binding to the cellular pre-mRNAs. The cap is then cleaved from the cellular pre-mRNA using a second viral protein, PB2. The short oligo cap is then added to the influenza +RNA strands, allowing its processing as messenger RNA by ribosomes. The +RNA strands also serve for synthesis of -RNA strands for new virions.

The RNA synthesis and its assembly with the nucleoprotein takes place in the cell nucleus, the synthesis of proteins takes place in the cytoplasm. The assembled virion cores leave the nucleus and migrate towards the cell membrane, with patches of viral transmembrane proteins (hemagglutinin, neuraminidase and M2 proteins) and an underlying layer of the M1 protein, and bud through these patches, releasing finished enveloped viruses into the extracellular fluid.

Avian Influenza

Wild fowl act as natural asymptomatic carriers of Influenza A viruses. Prior to the current H5N1 epizootic, strains of Influenza A virus had been demonstrated to be transmitted from wild fowl to only birds, pigs, horses, seals, whales and humans; and only between humans and pigs and between humans and domestic fowl; and not other pathways such as domestic fowl to horse.

Wild aquatic birds are the natural hosts for a large variety of influenza A viruses. Occasionally viruses are transmitted from these birds to other species and may then cause devastating outbreaks in domestic poultry or give rise to human influenza pandemics.

H5N1 has been shown to be transmitted to tigers, leopards, and domestic cats that were fed uncooked domestic fowl (chickens) with the virus. H3N8 viruses from horses have crossed over and caused outbreaks in dogs. Laboratory mice have been infected successfully with a variety of avian flu genotypes.

Influenza A viruses spread in the air and in manure and survives longer in cold weather. It can also be transmitted by contaminated feed, water, equipment and clothing; however, there is no evidence that the virus can survive in well-cooked meat. Symptoms in animals vary, but virulent strains can cause death within a few days.

> "Highly pathogenic avian influenza virus is on every top ten list available for potential agricultural bioweapon agents".

Avian influenza viruses that the OIE and others test for in order to control poultry disease include: H5N1, H7N2, H1N7, H7N3, H13N6, H5N9, H11N6, H3N8, H9N2, H5N2, H4N8, H10N7, H2N2, H8N4, H14N5, H6N5, H12N5 and others.

Known Outbreaks of Highly Pathogenic Flu in Poultry 1959-2003

Year	*Area*	*Affected*	*Subtype*
1959	Scotland	chicken	H5N1
1963	England	turkey	H7N3
1966	Ontario (Canada)	turkey	H5N9
1976	Victoria (Australia)	chicken	H7N7
1979	Germany	chicken	H7N7
1979	England	turkey	H7N7
1983	Pennsylvania (USA)*	chicken, turkey	H5N2
1983	Ireland	turkey	H5N8
1985	Victoria (Australia)	chicken	H7N7
1991	England	turkey	H5N1
1992	Victoria (Australia)	chicken	H7N3
1994	Queensland (Australia)	chicken	H7N3
1994	Mexico*	chicken	H5N2
1994	Pakistan*	chicken	H7N3
1997	New South Wales (Australia)	chicken	H7N4
1997	Hong Kong (China)*	chicken	H5N1
1997	Italy	chicken	H5N2
1999	Italy*	turkey	H7N1
2002	Hong Kong (China)	chicken	H5N1
2002	Chile	chicken	H7N3
2003	Netherlands*	chicken	H7N7

**Outbreaks with significant spread to numerous farms, resulting in great economic losses. Most other outbreaks involved little or no spread from the initially infected farms.*

1979: "More than 400 harbour seals, most of them immature, died along the New England coast between December 1979 and October 1980 of acute pneumonia associated with influenza virus, A/Seal/Mass/1/180 (H7N7)."

1995: "Vaccinated birds can develop asymptomatic infections that allow virus to spread, mutate, and recombine

(ProMED-mail, 2004j). Intensive surveillance is required to detect these "silent epidemics" in time to curtail them. In Mexico, for example, mass vaccination of chickens against epidemic H5N2 influenza in 1995 has had to continue in order to control a persistent and evolving virus (Lee *et al.*, 2004)."

1997: "Influenza A viruses normally seen in one species sometimes can cross over and cause illness in another species. For example, until 1997, only H1N1 viruses circulated widely in the US pig population. However, in 1997, H3N2 viruses from humans were introduced into the pig population and caused widespread disease among pigs. Most recently, H3N8 viruses from horses have crossed over and caused outbreaks in dogs."

2000: "In California, poultry producers kept their knowledge of a recent H6N2 avian influenza outbreak to themselves due to their fear of public rejection of poultry products; meanwhile, the disease spread across the western United States and has since become endemic."

2003: In Netherlands H7N7 influenza virus infection broke out in poultry on several farms.

2004: In North America, the presence of avian influenza strain H7N3 was confirmed at several poultry farms in British Columbia in February 2004. As of April 2004, 18 farms had been quarantined to halt the spread of the virus.

2005: Tens of millions of birds died of H5N1 influenza and hundreds of millions of birds were culled to protect humans from H5N1. H5N1 is endemic in birds in South East Asia and represents a long term pandemic threat.

2006: H5N1 spreads across the globe killing hundreds of millions of birds and over 100 people causing a significant H5N1 impact from both actual deaths and predicted possible deaths.

Swine Flu

Swine flu (or "pig influenza") refers to a subset of Orthomyxoviridae that create influenza in pigs and are endemic in pigs. The species of Orthomyxoviridae that can cause flu in pigs are Influenza A virus and Influenza C virus but not all genotypes of these two species infect pigs. The known subtypes of Influenza A virus that create influenza in pigs and are endemic in pigs are H1N1, H1N2, H3N1 and H3N2.

Horse Flu

Horse flu (or "Equine influenza") refers to varieties of Influenza A virus that affect horses. Horse 'flu viruses were only isolated in 1956. There are two main types of virus called equine-1 (H7N7) which commonly affects horse heart muscle and equine-2 (H3N8) which is usually more severe.

Dog Flu

Dog flu (or "canine influenza") refers to varieties of Influenza A virus that affect dogs. The equine influenza virus H3N8 was found to infect and kill greyhound race dogs that had died from a respiratory illness at a Florida racetrack in January 2004.

H3N8

H3N8 is now endemic in birds, horses and dogs.

4

Human Influenza Virus

Different Virus

"Human influenza virus" usually refers to those subtypes that spread widely among humans. H1N1, H1N2, and H3N2 are the only known Influenza A virus subtypes currently circulating among humans.

Genetic factors in distinguishing between "human flu viruses" and "avian influenza viruses" include:

PB2: (RNA polymerase): Amino acid (or residue) position 627 in the PB2 protein encoded by the PB2 RNA gene. Until H5N1, all known avian influenza viruses had a Glu at position 627, while all human influenza viruses had a lysine.

HA: (hemagglutinin): Avian influenza HA bind alpha 2-3 sialic acid receptors while human influenza HA bind alpha 2-6 sialic acid receptors. Swine influenza viruses have the ability to bind both types of sialic acid receptors.

> "About 52 key genetic changes distinguish avian influenza strains from those that spread easily among people, according to researchers in Taiwan, who analysed the genes of more than 400 A type flu viruses." "How many mutations would make an avian virus capable of infecting humans efficiently, or how many mutations would render

an influenza virus a pandemic strain, is difficult to predict. We have examined sequences from the 1918 strain, which is the only pandemic influenza virus that could be entirely derived from avian strains. Of the 52 species-associated positions, 16 have residues typical for human strains; the others remained as avian signatures. The result supports the hypothesis that the 1918 pandemic virus is more closely related to the avian influenza A virus than are other human influenza viruses."

Human flu symptoms usually include fever, cough, sore throat, muscle aches, conjunctivitis and, in severe cases, severe breathing problems and pneumonia that may be fatal. The severity of the infection will depend to a large part on the state of the infected person's immune system and if the victim has been exposed to the strain before, and is therefore partially immune.

Highly pathogenic H5N1 avian influenza in a human is far worse, killing 50 per cent of humans that catch it. In one case, a boy with H5N1 experienced diarrhoea followed rapidly by a coma without developing respiratory or flu-like symptoms.

The Influenza A virus subtypes that have been confirmed in humans, ordered by the number of known human pandemic deaths, are:

- H1N1 caused "Spanish Flu" and the 2009 swine flu outbreak;
- H2N2 caused "Asian Flu" in the late-1950s;
- H3N2 caused "Hong Kong Flu" in the late-1960s;
- H5N1 considered a global influenza pandemic threat through its spread in the mid-2000s;
- H7N7 has unusual zoonotic potential;
- H1N2 is currently endemic in humans and pigs;
- H9N2, H7N2, H7N3, H5N2, H10N7.

H1N1

H1N1 is currently endemic in both human and pig populations. A variant of H1N1 was responsible for the Spanish flu pandemic that killed some 50 million to 100 million people worldwide over about a year in 1918 and 1919. Another variant was named a pandemic threat in the 2009 swine flu outbreak. Controversy arose in October, 2005, after the H1N1 genome was published in the journal, *Science*, because of fears that this information could be used for bioterrorism.

> "When he compared the 1918 virus with today's human flu viruses, Dr. Taubenberger noticed that it had alterations in just 25 to 30 of the virus's **4,400** amino acids. Those few changes turned a bird virus into a killer that could spread from person to person."

H2N2

The Asian Flu was a pandemic outbreak of H2N2 avian influenza that originated in China in 1957, spread worldwide that same year during which a influenza vaccine was developed, lasted until 1958 and caused between one and four million deaths.

H3N2

H3N2 is currently endemic in both human and pig populations. It evolved from H2N2 by antigenic shift and caused the Hong Kong Flu pandemic of 1968 and 1969 that killed up to 750,000. "An early-onset, severe form of influenza A H3N2 made headlines when it claimed the lives of several children in the United States in late-2003."

The dominant strain of annual flu in January 2006 is H3N2. Measured resistance to the standard antiviral drugs amantadine and rimantadine in H3N2 has increased from 1 per cent in 1994 to 12 per cent in 2003 to 91 per cent in 2005.

> "Contemporary human H3N2 influenza viruses are now endemic in pigs in southern China and can reassort with avian H5N1 viruses in this intermediate host."

H5N1

H5N1 is the world's major influenza pandemic threat.

H7N7

H7N7 has unusual zoonotic potential. In 2003 in Netherlands 89 people were confirmed to have H7N7 influenza virus infection following an outbreak in poultry on several farms. One death was recorded.

H1N2

H1N2 is currently endemic in both human and pig populations. The new H1N2 strain appears to have resulted from the reassortment of the genes of the currently circulating influenza H1N1 and H3N2 subtypes. The hemagglutinin protein of the H1N2 virus is similar to that of the currently circulating H1N1 viruses and the neuraminidase protein is similar to that of the current H3N2 viruses.

H9N2

Low pathogenic avian influenza A (H9N2) infection was confirmed in 1999, in China and Hong Kong in two children, and in 2003 in Hong Kong in one child. All three fully recovered.

H7N2

One person in New York in 2003 and one person in Virginia in 2002 were found to have serologic evidence of infection with H7N2. Both fully recovered.

H7N3

In North America, the presence of avian influenza strain H7N3 was confirmed at several poultry farms in British Columbia in February 2004. As of April 2004, 18 farms had been quarantined to halt the spread of the virus. Two cases of humans with avian influenza have been confirmed in that region. "Symptoms included conjunctivitis and mild influenza-like illness." Both fully recovered.

H5N2

Japan's Health Ministry said Jan., 2006 that poultry farm workers in Ibaraki prefecture may have been exposed to H5N2 in 2005. The H5N2 antibody titers of paired sera of 13 subjects increased fourfold or more.

H10N7

In 2004 in Egypt H10N7 was reported for the first time in humans. It caused illness in two infants in Egypt. One child's father is a poultry merchant.

Evolution of Disease

Taubenberger says:

"All influenza A pandemics since [the Spanish flu pandemic], and indeed almost all cases of influenza A worldwide (excepting human infections from avian viruses such as H5N1 and H7N7), have been caused by descendants of the 1918 virus, including "drifted" H1N1 viruses and reassorted H2N2 and H3N2 viruses. The latter are composed of key genes from the 1918 virus, updated by subsequently incorporated avian influenza genes that code for novel surface proteins, making the 1918 virus indeed the "mother" of all pandemics.

Researchers from the National Institutes of Health used data from the Influenza Genome Sequencing Project and concluded that during the ten-year period examined most of the time the hemagglutinin gene in H3N2 showed no significant excess of mutations in the antigenic regions while an increasing variety of strains accumulated. This resulted in one of the variants eventually achieving higher fitness, becoming dominant, and in a brief interval of rapid evolution rapidly sweeping through the population and eliminating most other variants.

Influenzavirus B

Influenzavirus B is a genus in the virus family Orthomyxoviridae. The only species in this genus is called "Influenza B virus".

Influenza B viruses are only known to infect humans and seals, giving them influenza. This limited host range is apparently responsible for the lack of Influenzavirus B caused influenza pandemics in contrast with those caused by the morphologically similar Influenzavirus A as both mutate by both genetic drift and reassortment.

Further diminishing the impact of this virus "in man, influenza B viruses evolve slower than A viruses and faster than C viruses". Influenzavirus B mutates at a rate 2-3 times lower than type A. However, influenza B mutates enough that lasting immunity is not possible. For example at the US's Food and Drug Administration's (FDA) Centre for Biologics Evaluation and Research's Vaccines and Related Biological Products Advisory Committee's 101st meeting of February 16, 2005, an extensive discussion and vote was held concerning next year's flu vaccine virus selection including which influenza B strain to use in the formulation of the flu vaccine:

> "For Influenza B, the question was asked: are there new strains present? And the answer was yes, and in 2004, the majority of the viruses were similar to a strain called B/Shanghai/361/2002, which is from the so-called B/Yamagata/1688 hemagglutinin lineage. That lineage was not the one that was being used in the vaccine that was current last year. In a minority of the strains that were found during the epidemiological studies were similar to the strain that was in the vaccine for last year, which was B/Hong Kong/330/2001, which belongs to the HA lineage that we represent with the strain B/Victoria/287. In answer to the question were these new viruses spreading, the answer, of course, is definitely yes. The Fujian-like viruses had become widespread around the world and were predominant everywhere, and these B/Shanghai-like strains at the time we were holding this meeting in February were predominant not only in North America and the United States, but also in Asia and Europe."

Morphology

The Influenza B virus capsid is enveloped while its virion consists of an envelope, a matrix protein, a nucleoprotein complex, a nucleocapsid, and a polymerase complex. It is sometimes spherical and sometimes filamentous. Its 500 or so surface projections are made of hemagglutinin and neuraminidase.

Nucleic Acid

The Influenza B virus genome is 14648 nucleotides long and consists of eight segments of linear negative-sense, single-stranded RNA. The multipartite genome is encapsidated, each segment in a separate nucleocapsid, and the nucleocapsids are surrounded by one envelope.

Influenzavirus C

Influenzavirus C is a genus in the virus family Orthomyxoviridae, which includes those viruses which cause influenza. The only species in this genus is called "Influenza C virus".

Influenza C viruses are known to infect humans and pigs, giving them influenza. Flu due to the type C species is rare compared to types A or B, but can be severe and can cause local epidemics.

Types A and B have 8 RNA segments and encode 11 proteins. Subtype C has 7 RNA segments and encodes 9 proteins.

Infectious Salmon Anaemia Virus

Infectious salmon anaemia or anaemia (ISA) is a viral disease of Atlantic Salmon (*Salmo salar*) that affects fish farms in Canada, Norway, Scotland and Chile, causing severe losses to infected farms.

The aetiological agent of ISA is the infectious salmon anaemia virus (ISAV). ISAV, a RNA virus, is the only species in the genus "Isavirus" which is in the family Orthomyxoviridae.

Pathology

As the name implies, it causes severe anaemia of infected fish. Unlike mammals, the red blood cells of fish have DNA, and can become infected with viruses. The fish develop pale gills, and may swim close to the water surface, gulping for air. However, the disease can also develop without the fish showing any external signs of illness, the fish maintain a normal appetite, and then they suddenly die.

The disease can progress slowly throughout an infected farm and, in the worst cases, death rates may approach 100 per cent. Post-mortem examination of the fish has shown a wide range of causes of death. The liver and spleen may be swollen, congested or partially already dead. The circulatory system may stop working, and the blood may be contaminated with dead blood cells. Red blood cells still present often burst easily and the numbers of immature and damaged blood cells are increased.

Infectious salmon anaemia appears to be most like influenza viruses. Its mode of transfer and the natural reservoirs of infectious salmon anaemia virus are not fully understood. Apart from Atlantic salmon, both sea-run Brown trout (*Salmo trutta*) and Rainbow trout (*Onchorhyncus mykiss*) can be infected, but do not become sick, so it is thought possible that these species may act as important carriers and reservoirs of the virus.

Epidemiology

Prevalence: In the autumn of 1984, a new disease was observed in Atlantic salmon being farmed along the southwest coast of Norway. The disease, which was named Infectious salmon anaemia, spread slowly. By June 1988 it had become sufficiently widespread and serious to require the Norwegian Ministry of Agriculture, Fisheries and Food to declare it a notifiable disease.

In the summer of 1996, a new disease appeared in Atlantic salmon being farmed in New Brunswick, Canada. The death rate of the fish on affected farms was very high and, following extensive scientific examination of the victims, the disease was named "haemorrhagic kidney syndrome." Although the source and distribution of this disease was not known, the results of studies by Norwegian and Canadian scientists showed conclusively that the same virus was responsible for both infectious salmon anaemia and haemorrhagic kidney syndrome.

In May 1998, a salmon farm at Loch Nevis on the west coast of Scotland reported its suspicions of an outbreak of infectious salmon anaemia. The suspicions were confirmed, and by the end of the year, the disease had spread to an additional fifteen farms not only on the Scottish mainland but also on Skye and Shetland.

More recently (2008) there has been another outbreak of ISA in the Shetlands. ISA was detected in fish from just one site, which has since been harvested and will remain fallow. There is no evidence the disease has spread beyond this site, but two nearby SSF cages are under suspicion of carrying the disease and are also now clear of fish.

Chile has been dealing with a ISA outbreak over the last two years. This has spread nationwide and has caused havoc in what was a booming industry.

Transmission

Transmission of the virus has been demonstrated to occur by contact with infected fish or their secretions. Contact with equipment or people who have handled infected fish also transmits the virus. The virus can survive in seawater and, not surprisingly, a major risk factor for any uninfected farm is its proximity to an already infected farm.

More recently the sea louse, a small crustacean parasite that attacks the protective mucous, scales and skin of the salmon has been shown to carry the virus passively on its surface and in its digestive tract, although transmission of the disease by sea lice has not been demonstrated. It is not known whether the Infectious salmon anaemia virus can reproduce itself in the sea louse, although this is a remote possibility as viruses are usually very host specific unlike bacterial diseases that can replicate in ticks such as Lyme disease and Rocky Mountain Spotted Fever.

Control

ISA is major threat to the viability of salmon farming and is now the first of the diseases classified on List One of the European Commission's fish health regime. Amongst other measures, this requires the total eradication of the entire fish stock should an outbreak of the disease be confirmed on any farm. The economic and social consequences of both the disease and the measures used to control it are thus very far reaching.

Infectious salmon anaemia is currently regarded as a serious threat not only to farmed salmon, but also to dwindling stocks of wild salmon. Anecdotal evidence suggests that fish which survive the first infection become immune to the virus. Work is now underway to develop a vaccine against ISA. A recent report suggests that the North American virus may be slightly different from the Norwegian virus. This makes it unlikely that the sudden appearance of the disease, at least in Canada, was due to the importation of infected Norwegian fish. The possibility then is that a single vaccine might only be effective in a limited area and maybe only for a limited time.

Thogotovirus

Thogotovirus is a genus in the virus family Orthomyxoviridae. It can replicate in both tick cells and vertebrate cells and is usually transmitted by ticks.

Thogoto virus can be transmitted from infected to uninfected ticks when co-feeding on uninfected guinea pigs, even though the guinea pigs do not develop detectable viraemia.

THOV has been isolated from ticks in Africa and southern Europe. THOV is known to infect humans in natural settings. DHOV has been isolated from ticks in India, eastern Russia, Egypt, and southern Portugal. DHOV is able to infect humans, causing a febrile illness and encephalitis. THOV has 6 RNA segments and DHOV has 7.

5

Virus Characteristics

The virus is a novel strain of influenza from which human populations have been neither vaccinated nor naturally immunised. The CDC, after examining virus samples from suspected cases in Mexico, matched the strain with those from cases in Texas and California, and found no known linkages to either to animals or one another. It was also determined that the strain contained genes from four different flu viruses: North American swine influenza; North American avian influenza; human influenza; and two swine influenza viruses typically found in Asia and Europe. Further analysis showed that several of the proteins of the virus are most similar to strains that cause mild symptoms in humans, leading virologist Wendy Barclay to suggest on May 1 that the virus was unlikely to cause severe symptoms for most people.

Rate of Infection

According to the World Health Organisation, 66 countries had officially reported 19,723 cases of infection, including 117 deaths, as of June 3, 2009. Notably, the cases in Argentina, Australia and El Salvador more than doubled in each of WHO reporting cycle updates 41 and 42 (29 May and 1 June respectively). But according to CDC experts, however, the flu outbreak in the US is dying down in the country as a whole. As of May 30, Wisconsin had more cases than any other state:

1,430, but Wisconsin officials said that this was "nothing to worry about," pointing out that the higher numbers largely reflected the state's efficiency in testing suspected cases. Spokesman Seth Boffeli added that the Wisconsin cases had been relatively mild.

Some news reports indicated that the swine flu was spreading more widely than official figures indicate, with outbreaks in Europe and Asia following those of North and South America. According to the CDC, about one in 20 cases was being officially reported in the US. In the UK, according to virologist professor John Oxford, the virus may be 300 times more widespread than health authorities have said, with total infections estimated at 30,000 as of 24 May 09. Oxford's estimate comes as leading scientists are warning that estimates by the UK and other governments on the spread of the disease are "meaningless" and hiding its true extent. He also estimates that Japan may have approximately 30,000 cases. Professor Michael Osterholm, one of the world's top flu experts and an adviser to the US government, also called the official figures "meaningless," claiming that officials were not hiding cases, but were not hunting very hard to find them. Oxford also believes that thousands of people have caught the virus and "suffered only the most minor symptoms," or none at all, over the past weeks.

Although the United States was past its flu season, the Southern Hemisphere, where the virus had also spread, was entering the cold months when influenza cases increase. Jeffery Taubenberger, a National Institutes of Health researcher, stated that "I am loath to make predictions about what an influenza virus that mutates so rapidly will do," but he believes it will spread across the planet. Other experts concur, adding that "the new swine flu virus is almost certain to eventually infect every continent and country, although that may take years."

Virulence

Most fatalities have been in Mexico (72 per cent, as of June 5, 2009) where, according to the *New York Times*, the deaths from the illness have primarily been young, healthy adults. The WHO Rapid Pandemic Assessment Collaboration estimated the case fatality ratio in Mexico prior to mid-April to be 0.4 per cent. This is comparable to that of the 1957 Asian flu, a category 2 pandemic that killed approximately 1 to 4 million people.

By May 27, the CDC was reporting 6764 US cases in 47 states resulting in fourteen deaths, but noted that for the most part, the infections continue to be mild—similar to seasonal flu—and recovery is fairly quick.

Furthermore, analysis hasn't turned up any of the markers which scientists associate with the virulence of the 1918 "Spanish flu" virus, said Nancy Cox, head of the CDC's flu lab. In the state of New York, as of June 7, eight people have died from the outbreak, which has sparked "panic in schools, fear in hospitals and unease on the subways'," writes the *New York Daily News*.

Belinda Ostrowsky, a doctor at Montefiore Medical Centre's division of infectious diseases notes that the deaths so far are "a tiny fraction of the up to 2,000 New Yorkers who die every year from seasonal flu — with barely a public murmur." She adds, "When there's something that's new and unknown, it scares people."

Mutation Potential

On May 22, WHO chief Dr. Margaret Chan said that the virus must be closely monitored in the southern hemisphere, as it could mix with ordinary seasonal influenza and change in unpredictable ways. "In cases where the H1N1 virus is widespread and circulating within the general community, countries must expect to see more cases of severe and fatal infections," she said. "This is a subtle, sneaky virus."

This led other experts to become concerned that the new virus strain could mutate over the coming months. Guan Yi, a leading virologist from the University of Hong Kong, for instance, described the new H1N1 influenza virus as "very unstable", meaning it could mix and swap genetic material when exposed to other viruses.

During an interview he said "Both H1N1 and H5N1 are unstable so the chances of them exchanging genetic material are higher, whereas a stable (seasonal flu) virus is less likely to take on genetic material." The H5N1 virus is mostly limited to birds, but in rare cases when it infects humans it has a mortality rate of between 60 per cent to 70 per cent.

Experts worry about the emergence of a hybrid of the more virulent Asian-lineage HPAI (highly pathogenic avian influenza) A/H5N1 strain (media labelled "bird flu") with more human-transmissible Influenza A strains such as this novel 2009 swine-origin A/H1N1 strain (media labelled "swine flu"), especially since the H5N1 strain is and has been for years endemic in a variety of wild bird species in countries like China, Indonesia, Vietnam and Egypt.

Nor had federal health officials in the US dismissed the possibility that the worst was yet to come. "Far from it," Ann Schuchat of the CDC says, noting that the horrific 1918 flu epidemic, which killed millions in the United States alone, was preceded by a mild "herald" wave of cases in the spring, followed by devastating waves of illness in the fall. "That 1918 experience is in our minds," she said.

However, as of early-June, Schuchat reported "encouraging news" regarding any mutations to date, by announcing that samples of the virus from points around the globe are "genetically identical" to the strain found in the United States. "We have tested isolates from a wide geographic area, from the Americas, Europe, from Asia and New Zealand and we are not seeing variations in isolates from the genetic testing we do here."

Although cases have been relatively mild and patients recover quickly, health officials have warned that the virus could mutate into a more virulent form, putting greater numbers of people at risk.

Pandemic Potential

WHO Pandemic Influenza Phases (2009)

Phase	*Description*
Phase 1	No animal influenza virus circulating among animals have been reported to cause infection in humans.
Phase 2	An animal influenza virus circulating in domesticated or wild animals is known to have caused infection in humans and is therefore considered a specific potential pandemic threat.
Phase 3	An animal or human-animal influenza reassortant virus has caused sporadic cases or small clusters of disease in people, but has not resulted in human-to-human transmission sufficient to sustain community-level outbreaks.
Phase 4	Human to human transmission of an animal or human-animal influenza reassortant virus able to sustain community-level outbreaks has been verified.
Phase 5	The same identified virus has caused sustained community level outbreaks in two or more countries in one WHO region.
Phase 6	In addition to the criteria defined in Phase 5, the same virus has caused sustained community level outbreaks in at least one other country in another WHO region.
Post peak period	Levels of pandemic influenza in most countries with adequate surveillance have dropped below peak levels.
Post pandemic period	Levels of influenza activity have returned to the levels seen for seasonal influenza in most countries with adequate surveillance.

The WHO and CDC officials remained concerned that this outbreak might yet become a pandemic. WHO declared a Pandemic Alert Level of five, out of a maximum six, describing the degree to which the virus had been able to spread among humans, and using a Pandemic Severity Index, which predicts the number of fatalities if 30 per cent of the human population were infected. By the end of April, however, some scientists believed that the strain was unlikely to cause as many fatalities as earlier pandemics, and may not even be as damaging as a typical flu season. WHO Director General Margaret Chan, on May 22, continued to stop short of declaring the outbreak a "pandemic," by moving to alert level six, because of doubts fostered by its mild symptoms to that date along with fear that a pandemic "declaration would trigger mass panic" and be economically and politically damaging to many countries.

Defining a Pandemic

WHO is hesitating to raise its alert level and declare a phase 6 pandemic as the virus to date has caused generally mild symptoms. Raising it to level 6 would cause many countries to adopt a variety of plans, such as shutting borders, banning events and curtailing travel. It therefore wants to now factor in the "level of severity" in its pandemic alert system, whereas the existing system was partly based on earlier fears of a deadly bird flu pandemic with its much higher mortality rate. WHO has continued to debate new rules for the declaration as cases outside North America increased, suggesting that if it were to make the declaration it might "add a caveat indicating that the virus is not very lethal".

According to some experts, however, the outbreak was already a pandemic. Michael Osterholm, director of the Centre for Infectious Disease Research and Policy of the University of Minneapolis, feels that WHO's criteria for a pandemic has been met. While Britain's Health Secretary Alan Johnson requested that the disease's severity and other determinants, besides its geographic spread, need to be considered before the pandemic alert is raised to the highest of WHO's 6-level scale, since a move to phase 6 means that "emergency plans are instantly triggered around the globe." In addition, at phase 6, many pharmaceutical companies would switch from making seasonal flu shots to pandemic-specific vaccine, "potentially creating shortages of an immunisation to counter the normal winter flu season." Keiji Fukuda, WHO's assistant director general of health security and environment, states that a move to phase 6 would "signify a really substantial increase in risk of harm to people."

Osterholm felt that the primary concern should be "scientific integrity," stating, "If they want to change the definition, then go ahead. But don't say that we are not in phase 6 right now because we don't want to go there." Rather than redefine what constitutes a pandemic, he suggested that health officials should help people understand that the current threat may resemble the 1957 or 1968 pandemics, in which fewer than 4 million people died, rather than the 1918 Spanish flu, blamed for killing about 50 million.

Northern Hemisphere

As of early-June, the flu has been reported in more than 60 countries, mostly in the Northern Hemisphere, with the United States reporting the most cases — more than 10,000, including at least 18 deaths, according to the World Health Organisation.

As of May 30, 2009, seasonal flu is down, circulating at low levels; while the non-seasonal new H1N1 flu strain continues to spread and constitutes approximately 82 per cent of all influenza viruses reported to CDC in the last week of May 2009.

Southern Hemisphere

It is predicted that the virus will likely continue to spread worldwide as flu season ramps up in the Southern Hemisphere. As of June 6, Australia's second largest city, Melbourne, has been reported as the "swine flu capital of the world", with 1,011 cases in Victoria, mostly in Melbourne. In the entire country, confirmed cases have reached 1,207. However, according to professor Robert Booy from the University of Sydney, the reason Victoria has the highest per capita rate of swine flu in the world "may simply be down to Australia's tough testing regime," and "is probably the best in the world at detecting this influenza virus." As a result, he feels that the US and Mexico probably had more cases than have been reported, stating "I would be quite certain that there's ten to a hundredfold more cases in the US than are confirmed.

South America already has had more than 1000 cases, including two deaths in Chile. It will continue to be a threat south of the equator, where countries are entering the winter months and traditional flu season. Keiji Fukuda of WHO has stated than swine flu has already caused more infections than seasonal influenza at the start of Chile's winter flu season.

Symptoms and Expected Severity

The signs of infection with swine flu are similar to other forms of influenza, and include a fever, coughing, headaches, pain in the muscles or joints, sore throat, chills, fatigue and runny nose. Diarrhoea and vomiting have also been reported in some cases. People at higher risk of serious complications included people age 65 years and older, children younger than 5 years old, pregnant women, and people of any age with underlying medical conditions (such as asthma, diabetes, obesity, heart disease, or a weakened immune system (e.g., taking immunosuppressive medications or infected with HIV).

Most Cases Mild

Evidence mounted through May that the symptoms were milder than health officials initially feared. As of May 27, most of the 342 confirmed cases in New York City had been mild and there had been only 4 confirmed death from the virus. Similarly, Japan had reported 279, mostly mild flu cases, and no deaths, with the government reopening schools as of May 23, stating that the "virus should be considered more like a seasonal flu." In Mexico, where the outbreak began in April, Mexico City officials lowered their swine flu alert level as no new cases had been reported for a week.

Symptoms that may Require Medical Attention

Certain symptoms may require emergency medical attention. In children, for instance, those might include blue lips and skin, dehydration, rapid breathing, excessive sleeping and significant irritability that includes a lack of desire to be held. In adults, shortness of breath, pain in the chest or abdomen, sudden dizziness or confusion may indicate the need for emergency care. In both children and adults, persistent vomiting or the return of flu-like symptoms that include a fever and cough may require medical attention.

Underlying Conditions may Worsen Symptoms

WHO reported that almost one-half of the patients hospitalised in the United States had underlying conditions. "Among 30 patients hospitalised in California," stated the WHO report, "64 per cent had underlying conditions and two of five pregnant women developed complications, including spontaneous abortion and premature rupture of membranes." And on June 5, health officials in six states that reported deaths from swine flu said that all six patients had been diagnosed with other health problems.

However, doctors in New York suggested that people with "underlying conditions" who had flu symptoms should consult their doctors first. "Visiting an emergency room full of sick people may actually put them in more danger," wrote the *New York Times*. Dr. Steven J. Davidson, the chairman of emergency medicine department at Maimonides Medical Centre in Brooklyn commented "Like the asthmatics, we'd really prefer that pregnant women would stay away from the emergency departments."

Prevention and Treatment

Personal Hygiene: Recommendations to prevent infection by the virus consisted of the standard personal precautions against influenza. This included frequent washing of hands with soap and water or with alcohol-based hand sanitisers, especially after being out in public. The CDC advised not touching the mouth, nose or eyes, as these are primary modes of transmission. When coughing, they recommended coughing into a tissue and disposing of the tissue, then immediately washing the hands. Transmission was also reduced by disinfecting household surfaces with a disinfectant or a diluted bleach solution. CDC advised sick people to stay home from work, school, or social gatherings and to generally limit contact with others to avoid infecting them.

Surgical Masks: According to Dr. Laurene Mascola, director of acute communicable disease control for, the Los Angeles County Department of Public Health, "Masks may give people a false sense of security. You would have to wear it 100 per cent of the time that you are outside," she stated. According to mask manufacturer 3M, there are no "established exposure limits for biological agents" such as swine flu virus. The CDC recommended respirators classified as N95 for health care workers and caregivers with a respiratory infection. However, the CDC admits that they didn't know whether they would prevent swine flu infection.

Health officials in Los Angeles stated that facial masks aren't foolproof. "Once they get moist, they are no longer useful," Mascola said. "Your saliva is going to be pooling in that mask. That will make it not useful because germs will be able to permeate." She also points out that taking a mask on and off "contaminates it and makes it less useful," as well. It is effective "only for a 20-minute to a half-hour period," she said. "Even in those places during the SARS epidemic, they found hand-washing as effective as wearing masks."

Masks may, however, be of benefit in "crowded settings" or for people who are in close contact with infected persons. "Close contact" is defined as 1 metre or less by the World Health Organisation and 6 feet or less by the US Occupational Safety and Health Administration. Masks were not generally provided by airport security or airlines.

Home Treatment Remedies

The Mayo Clinic suggested a number of measures to help ease symptoms, including adequate hydration and rest, soup to ease congestion, and over-the-counter drugs to relieve pain.

The latter would relieve symptoms, but not treat the condition, and runs the risk of overdose or harm to children if used incorrectly. In general, most patients were expected to recover without requiring medical attention, with the exception of individuals with pre-existing or acquired complications.

Transmission

Person-to-person Sneezing and Coughing

Little data is available on the risk of airborne transmission specific to this particular virus. Mexican authorities distributed surgical masks to the general public. The UK Health Protection Agency considered facial masks unnecessary for the general public. Many authorities recommend the use of respirators by health-care workers in the vicinity of pandemic flu patients, particularly during aerosol generating procedures (e.g. intubation, chest physiotherapy, bronchoscopy).

Touching: Infection can be caused by touching something with flu viruses on it and then touching your mouth or nose. Hand washing was recommended to address this route of infection.

No Danger from Pork Consumption: The leading international health agencies stressed that the "influenza viruses are not known to be transmissible to people through eating processed pork or other food products derived from pigs."

Antiviral Drugs: According to the CDC, antiviral drugs can be given to treat those who become severely ill. These antiviral drugs are prescription medicines (pills, liquid or an inhaler) and act against influenza viruses, including H1N1 flu virus. There are two influenza antiviral medications that are recommended for use against H1N1 flu. The drugs that were used for treating H1N1 flu are called oseltamivir (Tamiflu) and zanamivir (Relenza). The CDC noted that as the H1N1 flu spreads, these antiviral drugs might become in short supply. Therefore, the drugs would be given first to those people who have been hospitalised or are at high risk of complications. The drugs worked best if given within 2 days of becoming ill, but might be given later if illness became severe or to those at a high risk for complications.

Tamiflu treatments have sometimes led to resistant human H1N1 viruses becoming established. Marie-Paule Kiely, WHO vaccine research director, said that it was "almost a given" that the new strain would undergo reassortment with resistant seasonal flu viruses and acquire some level of resistance. Other scientists agree that the virus will become resistant to the antiviral drug Tamiflu, noting that "a gene for Tamiflu resistance is now almost universal in seasonal H1N1 flus". If that happens, the "world's Tamiflu stockpiles will be all but worthless," writes the *New York Times*, and doctors would have to switch to the more expensive and harder to take, Relenza.

When buying these medications, some agencies warn against buying from online sources, with WHO estimating that half the drugs sold by online pharmacies without a physical address are counterfeit. Medical experts were also concerned that people "racing to grab up antiviral drugs just to feel safe" might eventually lead to the virus developing drug resistance. Partly as a result, experts suggested the medications should be reserved for only the very ill or people with severe immune deficiencies.

6

Epidemic and Pandemic Spread

As influenza is caused by a variety of species and strains of viruses, in any given year some strains can die out while others create epidemics, while yet another strain can cause a pandemic. Typically, in a year's normal two flu seasons (one per hemisphere), there are between three and five million cases of severe illness and up to 500,000 deaths worldwide, which by some definitions is a yearly influenza epidemic. Although the incidence of influenza can vary widely between years, approximately 36,000 deaths and more than 200,000 hospitalisations are directly associated with influenza every year in the United States. Roughly three times per century, a pandemic occurs, which infects a large proportion of the world's population and can kill tens of millions of people. Indeed, one study estimated that if a strain with similar virulence to the 1918 influenza emerged today, it could kill between 50 and 80 million people.

New influenza viruses are constantly evolving by mutation or by reassortment. Mutations can cause small changes in the hemagglutinin and neuraminidase antigens on the surface of the virus. This is called antigenic drift, which slowly creates an increasing variety of strains until one evolves that can infect people who are immune to the pre-existing strains. This new variant then replaces the older strains as it rapidly sweeps through the human population—often causing an epidemic. However, since the strains produced by drift will still be reasonably similar to the older strains, some people will still be immune to them. In contrast, when influenza viruses reassort, they acquire completely new antigens—for example by reassortment between avian strains and human strains; this is called antigenic shift. If a human influenza virus is produced that has entirely new antigens, everybody will be susceptible, and the novel influenza will spread uncontrollably, causing a pandemic. In contrast to this model of pandemics based on antigenic drift and shift, an alternative approach has been proposed where the periodic pandemics are produced by interactions of a fixed set of viral strains with a human population with a constantly changing set of immunities to different viral strains.

Prevention

Vaccination: Vaccination against influenza with an influenza vaccine is often recommended for high-risk groups, such as children and the elderly, or in people who have asthma, diabetes, or heart disease. Influenza vaccines can be produced in several ways; the most common method is to grow the virus in fertilized hen eggs. After purification, the virus is inactivated (for example, by treatment with detergent) to produce an inactivated-virus vaccine. Alternatively, the virus can be grown in eggs until it loses virulence and the avirulent virus given as a live vaccine. The effectiveness of these influenza vaccines are variable. Due to the high mutation rate of the virus, a particular influenza vaccine usually confers protection for no more than a few years. Every year, the World Health Organisation predicts which strains of the virus are most likely to be circulating in the next year, allowing pharmaceutical companies to develop vaccines that will provide the best immunity against these strains. Vaccines have also been developed to protect poultry from avian influenza. These vaccines can be effective against multiple strains and are used either as part of a preventative strategy, or combined with culling in attempts to eradicate outbreaks.

It is possible to get vaccinated and still get influenza. The vaccine is reformulated each season for a few specific flu strains but cannot possibly include all the strains actively infecting people in the world for that season. It takes about six months for the manufacturers to formulate and produce the millions of doses required to deal with the seasonal epidemics; occasionally, a new or overlooked strain becomes prominent during that time and infects people although they have been vaccinated (as by the H3N2 Fujian flu in the 2003–2004 flu season). It is also possible to get infected just before vaccination and get sick with the very strain that the vaccine is supposed to prevent, as the vaccine takes about two weeks to become effective.

The 2006–2007 season was the first in which the CDC had recommended that children younger than 59 months receive the annual influenza vaccine. Vaccines can cause the immune system to react as if the body were actually being infected, and general infection symptoms (many cold and flu symptoms are just general infection symptoms) can appear, though these symptoms are usually not as severe or long-lasting as influenza. The most dangerous side-effect is a severe allergic reaction to either the virus material itself or residues from the hen eggs used to grow the influenza; however, these reactions are extremely rare.

Infection Control

Good personal health and hygiene habits, like hand washing, avoiding spitting, and covering the nose and mouth when sneezing or coughing, are reasonably effective in reducing influenza transmission. In particular, hand-washing with soap and water, or with alcohol-based hand rubs, is very effective at inactivating influenza viruses. These simple personal hygiene precautions are recommended as the main way of reducing infections during pandemics. Although face masks might help prevent transmission when caring for the sick, evidence of beneficial effects is mixed in the community.

Since influenza spreads through both aerosols and contact with contaminated surfaces, surface sanitising may help prevent some infections. Alcohol is an effective sanitiser against influenza viruses, while quaternary ammonium compounds can be used with alcohol so that the sanitising effect lasts for longer. In hospitals, quaternary ammonium compounds and bleach are used to sanitise rooms or equipment that have been occupied by patients with influenza symptoms. At home, this can be done effectively with a diluted chlorine bleach.

During past pandemics, closing schools, churches and theatres slowed the spread of the virus but did not have a large effect on the overall death rate. It is uncertain if reducing public gatherings, by for example closing schools and workplaces, will reduce transmission since people with influenza may just be moved from one area to another; such measures would also be difficult to enforce and might be unpopular. When small numbers of people are infected, isolating the sick might reduce the risk of transmission.

Treatment

People with the flu are advised to get plenty of rest, drink plenty of liquids, avoid using alcohol and tobacco and, if necessary, take medications such as paracetamol (acetaminophen) to relieve the fever and muscle aches associated with the flu. Children and teenagers with flu symptoms (particularly fever) should avoid taking aspirin during an influenza infection (especially influenza type B), because doing so can lead to Reye's syndrome, a rare but potentially fatal disease of the liver. Since influenza is caused by a virus, antibiotics have no effect on the infection; unless prescribed for secondary infections such as bacterial pneumonia. Antiviral medication can be effective, but some strains of influenza can show resistance to the standard antiviral drugs.

The two classes of antiviral drugs used against influenza are neuraminidase inhibitors and M2 protein inhibitors (adamantane derivatives). Neuraminidase inhibitors are currently preferred for flu virus infections since they are less toxic and more effective. The CDC recommended against using M2 inhibitors during the 2005–06 influenza season due to high levels of drug resistance.

Neuraminidase Inhibitors

Antiviral drugs such as oseltamivir (trade name Tamiflu) and zanamivir (trade name Relenza) are neuraminidase inhibitors that are designed to halt the spread of the virus in the body. These drugs are often effective against both influenza A and B. The Cochrane Collaboration reviewed these drugs and concluded that they reduce symptoms and complications. Different strains of influenza viruses have differing degrees of resistance against these antivirals, and it is impossible to predict what degree of resistance a future pandemic strain might have.

M2 Inhibitors (adamantanes)

The antiviral drugs amantadine and rimantadine block a viral ion channel (M2 protein) and prevent the virus from infecting cells. These drugs are sometimes effective against influenza A if given early in the infection but are always ineffective against influenza B because B viruses do not possess M2 molecules. Measured resistance to amantadine and rimantadine in American isolates of H3N2 has increased to 91 per cent in 2005. This high level of resistance may be due to the easy availability of amantadines as part of over-the-counter cold remedies in countries such as China and Russia, and their use to prevent outbreaks of influenza in farmed poultry.

Research: Research on influenza includes studies on molecular virology, how the virus produces disease (pathogeneses), host immune responses, viral genomics, and how the virus spreads (epidemiology). These studies help in developing influenza countermeasures; for example, a better understanding of the body's immune system response helps vaccine development, and a detailed picture of how influenza invades cells aids the development of antiviral drugs. One important basic research programme is the Influenza Genome Sequencing Project, which is creating a library of influenza sequences; this library should help clarify which factors make one strain more lethal than another, which genes most affect immunogenicity, and how the virus evolves over time.

Research into new vaccines is particularly important, as current vaccines are very slow and expensive to produce and must be reformulated every year. The sequencing of the influenza genome and recombinant DNA technology may accelerate the generation of new vaccine strains by allowing scientists to substitute new antigens into a previously developed vaccine strain. New technologies are also being developed to grow viruses in cell culture, which promises higher yields, less cost, better quality and surge capacity. Research on a universal influenza A vaccine, targeted against the external domain of the transmembrane viral M2 protein (M2e), is being done at the University of Ghent by Walter Fiers, Xavier Saelens and their team and has now successfully concluded Phase I clinical trials.

A number of biologics, therapeutic vaccines and immunobiologics are also being investigated for treatment of infection caused by viruses. Therapeutic biologics are designed to activate the immune response to virus or antigens. Typically, biologics do not target metabolic pathways like antiviral drugs, but stimulate immune cells such as lymphocytes, macrophages, and/or antigen presenting cells, in an effort to drive an immune response towards a cytotoxic effect against the virus. Influenza models, such as murine influenza, are convenient models to test the effects of prophylactic and therapeutic biologics. For example, Lymphocyte T-Cell Immune Modulator inhibits viral growth in the murine model of influenza.

Infection in Animals

Influenza infects many animal species, and transfer of viral strains between species can occur. Birds are thought to be the main animal reservoirs of influenza viruses. Sixteen forms of hemagglutinin and nine forms of neuraminidase have been identified. All known subtypes (HxNy) are found in birds, but many subtypes are endemic in humans, dogs, horses, and pigs; populations of camels, ferrets, cats, seals, mink, and whales also show evidence of prior infection or exposure to influenza. Variants of flu virus are sometimes named according to the species the strain is endemic in or adapted to. The main variants named using this convention are: Bird Flu, Human Flu, Swine Flu, Horse Flu and Dog Flu. (Cat flu generally refers to Feline viral rhinotracheitis or Feline calicivirus and not infection from an influenza virus.) In pigs, horses and dogs, influenza symptoms are similar to humans, with cough, fever and loss of appetite. The frequency of animal diseases are not as well-studied as human infection, but an outbreak of influenza in harbour seals caused approximately 500 seal deaths off the New England coast in 1979-1980. On the other hand, outbreaks in pigs are common and do not cause severe mortality.

Bird Flu

Flu symptoms in birds are variable and can be unspecific. The symptoms following infection with low-pathogenicity avian influenza may be as mild as ruffled feathers, a small reduction in egg production, or weight loss combined with minor respiratory disease. Since these mild symptoms can make diagnosis in the field difficult, tracking the spread of avian influenza requires laboratory testing of samples from infected birds. Some strains such as Asian H9N2 are highly virulent to poultry and may cause more extreme symptoms and significant mortality. In its most highly pathogenic form, influenza in chickens and turkeys produces a sudden appearance of severe symptoms and almost 100 per cent mortality within two days. As the virus spreads rapidly in the crowded conditions seen in the intensive farming of chickens and turkeys, these outbreaks can cause large economic losses to poultry farmers.

An avian-adapted, highly pathogenic strain of H5N1 [called HPAI A(H5N1), for "highly pathogenic avian influenza virus of type A of subtype H5N1"] causes H5N1 flu, commonly known as "avian influenza" or simply "bird flu", and is endemic in many bird populations, especially in South East Asia. This Asian lineage strain of HPAI A(H5N1) is spreading globally. It is epizootic (an epidemic in non-humans) and panzootic (a disease affecting animals of many species, especially over a wide area), killing tens of millions of birds and spurring the culling of hundreds of millions of other birds in an attempt to control its spread. Most references in the media to "bird flu" and most references to H5N1 are about this specific strain.

At present, HPAI A(H5N1) is an avian disease, and there is no evidence suggesting efficient human-to-human transmission of HPAI A(H5N1). In almost all cases, those infected have had extensive physical contact with infected birds. In the future, H5N1 may mutate or reassort into a strain capable of efficient human-to-human transmission. The exact changes that are required for this to happen are not well understood. However, due to the high lethality and virulence of H5N1, its endemic presence, and its large and increasing biological host reservoir, the H5N1 virus was the world's pandemic threat in the 2006–07 flu season, and billions of dollars are being raised and spent researching H5N1 and preparing for a potential influenza pandemic.

Swine Flu

In pigs swine influenza produces fever, lethargy, sneezing, coughing, difficulty breathing and decreased appetite. In some cases the infection can cause abortion. Although mortality is usually low, the virus can produce weight loss and poor growth, causing economic loss to farmers. Infected pigs can lose up to 12 pounds of body weight over a 3 to 4 week period. Direct transmission of an influenza virus from pigs to humans is occasionally possible (this is called zoonotic swine flu). In all, 50 human cases are known to have occurred since the virus was identified in the mid-20th century, which have resulted in six deaths.

In 2009 an outbreak of influenza A virus subtype H1N1 occurred in Mexico. The virus is being commonly referred to as "swine flu", but there is no evidence of transmission from pigs to people, instead the virus is spreading from person to person. This strain is a reassortment of several strains of H1N1 that are usually found separately, in humans, birds, and pigs. It was first identified in the town of Perote in the State of Veracruz and in the City of Oaxaca, in Mexico, in March to April 2009.

Twenty six deaths have been conclusively proved to be due to this strain as they are the only ones officially recognised by the WHO as being clearly caused by this virus. The Mexican government introduced emergency measures, and sparked a coordinated international effort to contain the outbreak, which involved quarantine measures, restrictions in travel and stockpiling of treatments.

This outbreak prompted the World Health Organisation, on April 26, 2009 to declare the world one step closer to a pandemic, by raising the pandemic alert level from 3 to 4. Phase 4 refers to when there are small clusters—e.g., <25 human cases lasting <2 weeks with limited human-to-human transmission, but when spread is highly localised, which suggests the virus has not adapted well to humans. On Wednesday 29 April the WHO raised the pandemic risk scale from 4 to 5, one below pandemic phase.

7

Influenza Treatment

Treatments for influenza include a range of medications and therapies that are used in response to disease influenza. Treatments may either directly target the influenza virus itself; or instead they may just offer relief to symptoms of the disease, while the body's own immune system works to recover from infection.

The two main classes of antiviral drugs used against influenza are neuraminidase inhibitors, such as zanamivir and oseltamivir, or inhibitors of the viral M2 protein, such as amantadine and rimantadine.

These drugs can reduce the severity of symptoms if taken soon after infection and can also be taken to decrease the risk of infection. However, viral stains have emerged that show drug resistance to both classes of drug.

Symptomatic Treatment

The United States authority on disease prevention, the Centres for Disease Control and Prevention (CDC), recommends that persons suffering from influenza infections:

- Stay at home
- Get plenty of rest
- Drink a lot of liquids

- Do not smoke or drink alcohol
- Consider over-the-counter medications to relieve flu symptoms
- Consult a doctor early on for best possible treatment
- Remain alert for emergency warning signs

Warning signs are symptoms that indicate that the disease is becoming serious and needs immediate medical attention. These include:

- Difficulty breathing or shortness of breath
- Pain or pressure in the chest or abdomen
- Dizziness
- Confusion
- Severe or persistent vomiting

In children other warning signs include irritability, failing to wake up and interact, rapid breathing, and a blueish skin colour. Another warning sign in children is if the flu symptoms appear to resolve, but then reappear with fever and a bad cough.

Antiviral Drugs

Antiviral drugs directly target the viruses responsible for influenza infections. Generally, antiviral drugs work optimally when taken within a few days of the onset of symptoms. Certain drugs are used prophylactically, that is they are used in uninfected individuals to guard against infection.

Four licensed influenza antiviral agents are available in the United States: amantadine, rimantadine, zanamivir, and oseltamivir.

They are available through prescription only. These drugs fall into categories as either M2-inhibitors (admantane derivatives) or neuraminidase inhibitors as illustrated in the following table.

Antiviral Drugs to Treat Influenza

Class	*Effective Against*	*Drug Name (INN)*	*Brand Name*	*Year Approved*	*Manufacturer*
M2 inhibitors (adamantane derivatives)	Influenza A	Amantadine	Symmetrel	1976	Endo Pharmaceuticals
		Rimantadine	Flumadine	1994	Forest Laboratories
Neuraminidase inhibitors	Influenza A & B	Zanamivir	Relenza	1999	Glaxo SmithKline
		Oseltamivir	Tamiflu	1999	Hoffmann-La Roche

Note: Neuraminidase inhibitors are approved for prophylaxis use in children and adults.

In Russia and China a drug called arbidol is also used as a treatment. Testing of the drug has predominantly occurred in these countries and, although no clinical trials have been published demonstrating this is an effective drug, some data suggest that this could be a useful treatment for influenza.

Peramivir, an experimental anti-influenza drug, developed by BioCryst Pharmaceuticals has not yet been approved for sale in the United States.

Drug Resistance

Influenza viruses can show resistance to antiviral drugs. Like the development of bacterial antibiotic resistance, this can result from over-use of these drugs. For example, in the case of the amantadines treatment may lead to the rapid production of resistant viruses, and over-use of these drugs has probably contributed to the spread of resistance. In particular, this high-level of resistance may be due to the easy availability of amantadines as part of over-the-counter cold remedies in countries such as China and Russia, and their use to prevent outbreaks of influenza in farmed poultry.

On the other hand, a few strains resistant to neuraminidase inhibitors have emerged and circulated in the absence of much use of the drugs involved, and the frequency with which drug resistant strains appears shows little correlation with the level of use of these drugs. However, laboratory studies have shown that it is possible for the use of sub-optimal doses of these drugs as a prophylactic measure might contribute to the development of drug resistance.

During the United States 2005–2006 influenza season, increasing incidence of drug resistance by strain H3N2 to amantadine and rimantadine led the CDC to recommend oseltamivir as a prophylactic drug, and the use of either oseltamivir or zanamivir as treatment.

Over-the-counter Medication

Antiviral drugs are prescription-only medication in the United States. Readily available over-the-counter medications do not directly affect the disease, but they do provide relief from influenza symptoms, as illustrated in the table below.

OTC Medicines Provide Relief for Flu Symptoms

Symptom(s)	*OTC Medicine*
fever, aches, pains, sinus pressure, sore throat	analgesics
nasal congestion, sinus pressure	decongestants
sinus pressure, runny nose, watery eyes, cough	antihistamines
cough	cough suppressant
sore throat	local anesthetics

Children and teenagers with flu symptoms (particularly fever) should avoid taking aspirin as taking aspirin in the presence of influenza infection (especially Influenzavirus B) can lead to Reye's syndrome, a rare but potentially fatal disease of the liver.

Influenza Vaccine

The influenza vaccine is an annual vaccine to protect against the highly variable influenza virus.

Purpose and Benefits of Annual Flu Vaccination

> "Influenza vaccination is the most effective method for preventing influenza virus infection and its potentially severe complications."

An influenza epidemic emerges during each winter's flu season. In the United States alone an estimated 36,000 people die each year from influenza and accompanying opportunistic infections and complications. The economic costsin the US have been estimated at over $80 billion.

The number of annual influenza-related hospitalisations is many times the number of deaths. "The high costs of hospitalising young children for influenza creates a significant economic burden in the United States, underscoring the importance of preventive flu shots for children and the people with whom they have regular contact..."

In Canada, the National Advisory Committee on Immunisation, the group that advises the Public Health Agency of Canada, currently recommends that everyone aged 2 to 64 years be encouraged to receive annual influenza vaccination, and that children between the age of six and 24 months, and their household contacts, should be considered a high priority for the flu vaccine.

In the United States, the CDC recommends to clinicians that:

> In general, anyone who wants to reduce their chances of getting influenza can get vaccinated. Vaccination is especially important for people at higher risk of serious influenza complications or people who live with or care for people at higher risk for serious complications.

Vaccination against influenza is recommended for most members of high-risk groups who would be likely to suffer complications from influenza. Specific recommendations include all children and teenagers, from six months to 18 years; of age:

> In expanding the new upper age limit to 18 years, the aim is to reduce both the time children and parents lose from visits to paediatricians and missing school and the need for antibiotics for complications ...
>
> An added expected benefit would be indirect — to reduce the number of influenza cases among parents and other household members, and possibly spread to the general community.

In the event of exposure to H5N1-type (avian influenza), seasonal flu vaccine may also offer some protection against H5N1 infection.

Efficacy of Vaccine

Flu vaccines are available both as an injection of killed virus (or flu shot) and as nasal spray of live attenuated influenza virus (LAIV) (sold as FluMist in the United States). LAIV is not recommended for individuals under age 2 or over age 50.

Vaccine is effective against influenza, but not perfect. A study led by Dr. David K. Shay in February, 2008 reported that:

> "full immunisation against flu provided about a 75 per cent effectiveness rate in preventing hospitalisations from influenza complications in the 2005-6 and 2006-7 influenza seasons."

While no statistically significant advantage emerged for either LAIV or TIV (needle-injected vaccine) over the other in two trials among adults noted by the CDC, the benefit of influenza vaccination over non-vaccination were clear:

"One randomised, double-blind, placebo-controlled challenge study among 92 healthy adults aged 18–41 years assessed the efficacy of both LAIV and TIV in preventing influenza infection when challenged with wild-type strains that were antigenically similar to vaccine strains. The overall efficacy in preventing laboratory-documented influenza from all three influenza strains combined was 85 per cent and 71 per cent, respectively.

In a randomised, double-blind, placebo-controlled trial, conducted among young adults during an influenza season when the majority of circulating H3N2 viruses were antigenically drifted from that season's vaccine viruses, the efficacy of LAIV and TIV against culture-confirmed influenza was 57 per cent and 77 per cent, respectively.

The 57-77 per cent efficacy rate of the influenza vaccine is not universal, however. The group most vulnerable to the illness, the elderly, is also the least affected by the vaccine, with an average efficacy rate ranging from 40-50 per cent at age 65, and 15-30 per cent past age 70. There are multiple reasons behind this steep decline in vaccine efficacy, the most common of which are the declining immunological function and frailty associated with advanced age.

Neither the comparative advantages of LAIV in the first study nor the apparent advantages of needle-injected vaccine in the second rose to statistical significance. The added benefits of needle-injected vaccine in the second study "was based largely upon a difference in efficacy against influenza B."

LAIV may be comparatively more effective among children. In studies conducted before final approval for two-year olds and older children, FluMist demonstrated a definite immunological advantage over flu shots in this age group.

These studies demonstrate that vaccination can be a cost-effective counter-measure to seasonal outbreaks of influenza.

In most years (16 of the 19 years before 2007), the flu vaccine strains have been a good match for the circulating strains. In other flu seasons like that of 2007/2008, the match was less useful. But even a mis-matched vaccine can often provide some protection:

> ...Antibodies made in response to vaccination with one strain of influenza viruses can provide protection against different, but related strains. A

> less than ideal match may result in reduced vaccine effectiveness against the variant viruses, but it still can provide enough protection to prevent or lessen illness severity and prevent flu-related complications. In addition, it's important to remember that the influenza vaccine contains three virus strains so the vaccine can also protect against the other two viruses. For these reasons, even during seasons when there is a less than ideal match, CDC continues to recommend influenza vaccination. This is particularly important for people at high risk for serious flu complications and their close contacts.

Analysis of studies concluded that people over 65 who got flu shots were half as likely to die over the winter as their unvaccinated peers; this has become the consensus view. However, it has been pointed out that the number of flu deaths among elderly people in the US has remained at around 5 per cent of winter deaths from 1980 until 2005, although vaccination coverage increased from around 15 per cent in 1980 to around 70 per cent in 2005. Also the biggest supposed benefit from the flu shot occurred in the months *before* the flu season had started.

While accepting that vaccination reduced the risk of dying of flu, the analysis pointed out the need to develop better statistical methods for measuring the effectiveness of the flu vaccine.

History of the Flu Vaccine

Vaccines are used in both humans and non-humans. Human vaccine is meant unless specifically identified as a veterinary, poultry or livestock vaccine.

Influenza: The first influenza pandemic was recorded in 1580; since this time, various methods have been employed to eradicate its cause. The etiological cause of influenza, the orthomyxoviridae was finally discovered by the Medical Research Council (MRC) of the United Kingdom in 1933.

Known flu pandemics:

- 1889-90 — Asiatic (Russian) Flu, mortality rate said to be 0.75-1 death per 1000 possibly H2N2.
- 1900 — Possibly H3N8.
- 1918-20 – Spanish Flu, 500 million ill, at least 20-40 million died of H1N1.
- 1957-58 – Asian Flu, 1 to 1.5 million died of H2N2.
- 1968-69 – Hong Kong Flu, 3/4 to 1 million died of H3N2.

Flu Vaccine Origins and Development

In the world wide Spanish flu pandemic of 1918, "Physicians tried everything they knew, everything they had ever heard of, from the ancient art of bleeding patients, to administering oxygen, to developing new vaccines and sera (chiefly against what we now call *Hemophilus influenzae*—a name derived from the fact that it was originally considered the etiological agent—and several types of pneumococci). Only one therapeutic measure, transfusing blood from recovered patients to new victims, showed any hint of success."

In 1931, viral growth in embryonated hens' eggs was discovered, and in the 1940s, the US military developed the first approved inactivated vaccines for influenza, which were used in the Second World War (Baker 2002, Hilleman 2000). Greater advances were made in vaccinology and immunology, and vaccines became safer and mass-produced. Today, thanks to the advances of molecular technology, we are on the verge of making influenza vaccines through the genetic manipulation of influenza genes (Couch 1997, Hilleman 2002).

Flu Vaccine Acceptance

According to the CDC: "Influenza vaccination is the primary method for preventing influenza and its severe complications. [...] Vaccination is associated with reductions in influenza-related respiratory illness and physician visits among all age groups, hospitalisation and death among persons at high risk, otitis media among children, and work absenteeism among adults. Although influenza vaccination levels increased substantially during the 1990s, further improvements in vaccine coverage levels are needed".

The current egg-based technology for producing influenza vaccine was created in the 1950s. In the US swine flu scare of 1976, President Gerald Ford was confronted with a potential swine flu pandemic. The vaccination programme was plagued by delays and public relations problems, but about 24 per cent of the population was vaccinated by the time the programme was cancelled with much concern and doubt about flu vaccination.

Current Status: Influenza research includes molecular virology, molecular evolution, pathogeneses, host immune responses, genomics, and epidemiology. These help in developing influenza countermeasures such as vaccines, therapies and diagnostic tools. Improved influenza countermeasures require basic research on how viruses enter cells, replicate, mutate, evolve into new strains and induce an immune response. The Influenza Genome Sequencing Project is creating a library of influenza sequences that will help us understand what makes one strain more lethal than another, what genetic determinants most affect immunogenicity, and how the virus evolves over time. Solutions to limitations in current vaccine methods are being researched.

Today, we have the capability to produce 300 million doses of trivalent vaccine per year — enough for current epidemics in the Western world, but insufficient for coping with a pandemic.

Clinical Trials of Vaccines

A vaccine is assessed in terms of the reduction of the risk of disease produced by vaccination, its *efficacy*. In contrast, in the field, the *effectiveness* of a vaccine is the practical reduction in risk for an individual when they are vaccinated under real-world conditions. Measuring efficacy of influenza vaccines is relatively simple, as the immune response produced by the vaccine can be assessed in animal models, or the amount of antibody produced in vaccinated people can be measured, or most rigorously, by immunising adult volunteers and then challenging with virulent influenza virus.

In studies such as these, influenza vaccines showed high efficacy and produced a protective immune response. For ethical reasons, such challenge studies cannot be performed in the population most at risk from influenza – the elderly and young children. However, studies on the effectiveness of flu vaccines in the real world are uniquely difficult. The vaccine may not be matched to the virus in circulation; virus prevalence varies widely between years, and influenza is often confused with other flu-like illnesses.

Nevertheless, multiple clinical trials of both live and inactivated influenza vaccines have been performed and their results pooled and analysed in several recent meta-analyses. Studies on live vaccines have very limited data, but these preparations may be more effective than inactivated vaccines.

The meta-analyses examined the efficacy and effectiveness of inactivated vaccines in adults, children, and the elderly. In adults, vaccines show high efficacy against the targeted strains, but low effectiveness overall, so the benefits of vaccination are small, with a one-quarter reduction in risk of contracting influenza but no effect on the rate of hospitalisation. In children, vaccines again showed high efficacy, but low effectiveness in preventing "flu-like illness", in children under two the data are extremely limited, but vaccination appeared to confer no measurable benefit.

In the elderly, vaccination does not reduce the frequency of influenza, but may reduce pneumonia, hospital admission and deaths from influenza or pneumonia. The measured effectiveness of the vaccine in the elderly varies depending on whether the population studied is in residential care homes, or in the community, with the vaccine appearing more effective in an institutional environment. This apparent effect may be due to selection bias affecting the analysis of the data, or differences in diagnosis and surveillance.

Overall, the benefit of influenza vaccination is clearest in the elderly, with vaccination in children of questionable benefit. Vaccination of adults is not predicted to produce significant improvements in public health. The apparent contradiction between vaccines with high efficacy, but low effectiveness, may reflect the difficulty in diagnosing influenza under clinical conditions and the large number of strains circulating in the population.

Vaccination Recommendations: Various public health organisations have recommended that yearly influenza vaccination be routinely offered to patients at risk of complications of influenza:

- the elderly (UK recommendation is those aged 65 or above)
- patients with chronic lung diseases (asthma, COPD, etc.)
- patients with chronic heart diseases (congenital heart disease, chronic heart failure, ischaemic heart disease),
- patients with chronic liver diseases (including liver cirrhosis)
- patients with chronic renal diseases (such as the nephrotic syndrom)
- patients who are immunosuppressed (those with HIV or who are receiving drugs to suppress the immune system such as chemotherapy and long-term steroids) and their household contacts
- people who live together in large numbers in an environment where influenza can spread rapidly, such as prisons, nursing homes and dormitories
- health care workers (both to prevent sickness and to prevent spread to patients)
- pregnant women

In the United States a person aged 50–64 is nearly ten times more likely to die an influenza-associated death than a younger person, and a person over age 65 is over ten times more likely to die an influenza-associated death than the 50–64 age group. Vaccination of those over age 65 reduces influenza-associated death by about 50 per cent.

However, it is unlikely that the vaccine completely explains the results since elderly people who get vaccinated are probably more healthy and health-conscious than those who do not. Elderly participants randomised to a high-dose group (60 micrograms) had antibody levels 44 to 79 per cent higher than did those who received the normal dose of vaccine. Elderly volunteers receiving the higher dose were more likely to achieve protective levels of antibody.

As mortality is high among infants who contract influenza, the household contacts and caregivers of infants should be vaccinated to reduce the risk of passing an influenza infection to the infant.

Data from the years when Japan required annual flu vaccinations for school-aged children indicate that vaccinating children—the group most likely to catch and spread the disease—has a strikingly positive effect on reducing mortality among older people: one life saved for every 420 children who received the flu vaccine. This may be due to herd immunity or to direct causes, such as individual older people not being exposed to influenza. For example, retired grandparents often risk infection by caring for their sick grandchildren in households where the parents can't take time off work or are sick themselves.

Side Effects

Side effects of the inactivated/dead flu vaccine injection are:

- mild soreness,
- redness,
- death (very rare),

- swelling where the shot was given,
- fever,
- aches.

These problems usually begin soon after the injection, and last 1-2 days.

Side effects of the activated/live/LAIV flu nasal spray vaccine: Some children and adolescents 2-17 years of age have reported mild reactions, including:

- runny nose, nasal congestion or cough,
- fever,
- headache and muscle aches,
- wheesing,
- abdominal pain or occasional vomiting or diarrhoea.

Some adults 18-49 years of age have reported:

- runny nose or nasal congestion,
- sore throat,
- cough, chills, tiredness/weakness,
- headache.

Some injection-based flu vaccines intended for adults in the United States contain thiomersal. Despite some controversy in the media, the World Health Organisation has concluded that there is no evidence of toxicity from thimerosal in vaccines and no reason on grounds of safety to change to more-expensive single-dose administration.

Flu Vaccine Virus Selection

Each year, three strains are chosen for selection in that year's flu vaccination by the WHO Global Influenza Surveillance Network. The chosen strains are the H1N1, H3N2, and Type-B strains thought most likely to cause significant human suffering in the coming season.

> "The WHO Global Influenza Surveillance Network was established in 1952. The network comprises 4

> WHO Collaborating Centres (WHO CCs) and 112 institutions in 83 countries, which are recognised by WHO as WHO National Influenza Centres (NICs). These NICs collect specimens in their country, perform primary virus isolation and preliminary antigenic characterisation. They ship newly isolated strains to WHO CCs for high level antigenic and genetic analysis, the result of which forms the basis for WHO recommendations on the composition of influenza vaccine for the Northern and Southern Hemisphere each year."

The Global Influenza Surveillance Network's selection of viruses for the vaccine manufacturing process is based on its best estimate of which strains will be predominant the next year, amounting in the end to well-informed but fallible guesswork.

Flu Vaccine Manufacturing

Flu vaccine is usually grown in fertilized chicken eggs. Both types of flu vaccines are contraindicated for those with severe allergies to egg proteins and people with a history of Guillain-Barré syndrome.

On October 5, 2004, Chiron Corporation, a corporation contracted to deliver half of the expected flu vaccine for the United States and a significant portion to the UK, issued a press release that stated it was unable to dispense its stock for the 2004-2005 season, due to suspension of the corporation's license to produce the vaccine by the Medicines and Health care Products Regulatory Agency. However, the Centres for Disease Control and Prevention took swift action to enlist the help of other companies such as MedImmune and Sanofi Pasteur to supply vaccine in high-risk populations in the United States.

As of November 2007, both the conventional injection and the nasal spray are manufactured using chicken eggs. The European Union has also approved Optaflu, a vaccine produced by Novartis using vats of animal cells. This technique is expected to be more scalable and avoid problems with eggs, such as allergic reactions and incompatibility with strains that affect avians like chickens. A DNA-based vaccination, which is hoped to be even faster to manufacture, is currently in clinical trials, but has not yet been proven safe and effective. Research continues into the idea of a "universal" influenza vaccine (but no vaccine candidates have been announced) which would not need to be tailored to work on particular strains, but would be effective against a broad variety of influenza viruses.

H5N1: Vaccines have been formulated against several of the avian H5N1 influenza varieties. Vaccination of poultry against the ongoing H5N1 epizootic is widespread in certain countries. Some vaccines also exist for use in humans, and others are in testing, but none have been made available to civilian populations, nor produced in quantities sufficient to protect more than a tiny fraction of the Earth's population in the event that an H5N1 pandemic breaks out.

Three H5N1 vaccines for humans have been licensed as of June 2008:

- Sanofi Pasteur's vaccine approved by the United States in April 2007,
- GlaxoSmithKline's vaccine Pandemrix approved by the European Union in May 2008, and
- CSL Limited's vaccine approved by Australia in June 2008.

All are produced in eggs and would require many months to be altered to a pandemic version.

H5N1 continually mutates, meaning vaccines based on current samples of avian H5N1 cannot be depended upon to work in the case of a future pandemic of H5N1. While there can be some cross-protection against related flu strains, the best protection would be from a vaccine specifically produced for any future pandemic flu virus strain. Dr. Daniel Lucey, co-director of the Biohazardous Threats and Emerging Diseases graduate programme at Georgetown University, has made this point, "There is no H5N1 pandemic so there can be no pandemic vaccine." However, "pre-pandemic vaccines" have been created; are being refined and tested; and do have some promise both in furthering research and preparedness for the next pandemic. Vaccine manufacturing companies are being encouraged to increase capacity so that if a pandemic vaccine is needed, facilities will be available for rapid production of large amounts of a vaccine specific to a new pandemic strain.

Problems with H5N1 vaccine production include:

- lack of overall production capacity;
- lack of surge production capacity (it is impractical to develop a system that depends on hundreds of millions of 11-day old specialised eggs on a standby basis);
- the pandemic H5N1 might be lethal to chickens.

Annual Reformulation of Flu Vaccine

Each year the influenza virus changes and different strains become dominant. Due to the high mutation rate of the virus a particular vaccine formulation is effective for at most about a year. The World Health Organisation coordinates the contents of the vaccine each year to contain the most likely strains of the virus to attack the next year.

2002-2003 Season (Northern Hemisphere)

The vaccines produced for the 2002–2003 season use:

- an A/New Caledonia/20/1999-like(H1N1);
- an A/Moscow/10/1999-like(H3N2);
- a B/Hong Kong/330/2001-like viruses.

2003 Season (Southern Hemisphere)

The composition of influenza virus vaccines for use in the 2003 Southern Hemisphere influenza season recommended by the World Health Organisation was:

- an A/New Caledonia/20/99(H1N1)-like virus;
- an A/Moscow/10/99(H3N2)-like virus (The widely used vaccine strain is A/Panama/2007/99);

- a B/Hong Kong/330/2001-like virus (Some vaccine strains used were B/Shandong/7/97, B/Hong Kong/330/2001, B/Hong Kong/1434/2002).

2003-2004 Season (Northern Hemisphere)

The production of flu vaccine requires a lead time of about six months before the season. It is possible that by flu season a strain becomes common for which the vaccine does not provide protection. In the 2003-2004 season the vaccine was produced to protect against A/Panama, A/New Caledonia, and B/Hong Kong. A new strain, A/Fujian, was discovered after production of the vaccine started and vaccination gave only partial protection against this strain.

Nature magazine reported that the Influenza Genome Sequencing Project, using phylogenetic analysis of 156 H3N2 genomes, "explains the appearance, during the 2003-2004 season, of the 'Fujian/411/2002'-like strain, for which the existing vaccine had limited effectiveness" as due to an epidemiologically significant reassortment. "Through a reassortment event, a minor clade provided the haemagglutinin gene that later became part of the dominant strain after the 2002-2003 season. Two of our samples, A/New York/269/2003 (H3N2) and A/New York/32/2003 (H3N2), show that this minor clade continued to circulate in the 2003-2004 season, when most other isolates were reassortants."

According to the CDC: During the 2003-2004 influenza season, influenza A (H1), A (H3N2), and B viruses co-circulated worldwide, and influenza A (H3N2) viruses predominated. Several Asian countries reported widespread outbreaks of avian influenza A (H5N1) among poultry. In Vietnam and Thailand, these outbreaks were associated with severe illnesses and deaths among humans. In the United States, the 2003–2004 influenza season began earlier than most seasons, peaked in December, was moderately severe in terms of its impact on mortality, and was associated predominantly with influenza A (H3N2) viruses.

During September 28, 2003 – May 22, 2004, WHO and NREVSS collaborating laboratories in the United States tested

130,577 respiratory specimens for influenza viruses; 24,649 (18.9%) were positive. Of these, 24,393 (99.0%) were influenza A viruses, and 249 (1.0%) were influenza B viruses. Among the influenza A viruses, 7,191 (29.5%) were subtyped; 7,189 (99.9%) were influenza A (H3N2) viruses, and two (0.1%) were influenza A (H1) viruses. The proportion of specimens testing positive for influenza first increased to >10% during the week ending October 25, 2003 (week 43), peaked at 35.2 per cent during the week ending November 29 (week 48), and declined to <10 per cent during the week ending January 17, 2004 (week 2). The peak percentage of specimens testing positive for influenza during the previous four seasons had ranged from 23 per cent to 31 per cent and peaked during late-December to late-February.

As of June 15, 2004, CDC had antigenically characterised 1,024 influenza viruses collected by US laboratories since October 1, 2003: 949 influenza A (H3N2) viruses, three influenza A (H1) viruses, one influenza A (H7N2) virus, and 71 influenza B viruses. Of the 949 influenza A (H3N2) isolates characterised, 106 (11.2%) were similar antigenically to the vaccine strain A/Panama/2007/99 (H3N2), and 843 (88.8%) were similar to the drift variant, A/Fujian/411/2002 (H3N2). Of the three A (H1) isolates that were characterised, two were H1N1 viruses, and one was an H1N2 virus. The hemagglutinin proteins of the influenza A (H1) viruses were similar antigenically to the hemagglutinin of the vaccine strain A/New Caledonia/20/99. Of the 71 influenza B isolates that were characterised, 66 (93%) belonged to the B/Yamagata/16/88 lineage and were similar antigenically to B/Sichuan/379/99, and five (7%) belonged to the B/Victoria/2/87 lineage and were similar antigenically to the corresponding vaccine strain B/Hong Kong/330/2001.

H9N2: In December 2003, one confirmed case of avian influenza A (H9N2) virus infection was reported in a child aged five years in Hong Kong. The child had fever, cough, and nasal discharge in late-November, was hospitalised for two days, and fully recovered. The source of this child's H9N2 infection is unknown.

H5N1: During January–March 2004, a total of 34 confirmed human cases of avian influenza A (H5N1) virus infection were reported in Vietnam and Thailand. The cases were associated with severe respiratory illness requiring hospitalisation and a case-fatality proportion of 68 per cent (Vietnam: 22 cases, 15 deaths; Thailand: 12 cases, eight deaths). A substantial proportion of the cases were among children and young adults (i.e., persons aged 5–24 years). These cases were associated with widespread outbreaks of highly pathogenic H5N1 influenza among domestic poultry.

H7N3: During March 2004, health authorities in Canada reported two confirmed cases of avian influenza A (H7N3) virus infection in poultry workers who were involved in culling of poultry during outbreaks of highly pathogenic H7N3 on farms in the Fraser River Valley, British Columbia. One patient had unilateral conjunctivitis and nasal discharge, and the other had unilateral conjunctivitis and headache. Both illnesses resolved without hospitalisation.

H7N2: During the 2003–2004 influenza season, a case of avian influenza A (H7N2) virus infection was detected in an adult male from New York, who was hospitalised for upper and lower respiratory tract illness in November 2003. Influenza A (H7N2) virus was isolated from a respiratory specimen from the patient, whose acute symptoms resolved. The source of this person's infection is unknown.

2004 Season (Southern Hemisphere): The composition of influenza virus vaccines for use in the 2004 Southern Hemisphere influenza season recommended by the World Health Organisation was:

- an A/New Caledonia/20/99(H1N1)-like virus
- an A/Fujian/411/2002(H3N2)-like virus (A/Kumamoto/102/2002 and A/Wyoming/3/2003 were egg-grown A/Fujian/411/2002-like viruses)
- a B/Hong Kong/330/2001-like virus (B/Shandong/7/97, B/Hong Kong/330/2001 and B/Hong Kong/1434/

2002 were among those used at the time. B/Brisbane/32/2002 was also available.)

2004-2005 Season (Northern Hemisphere)

According to the CDC: On the basis of antigenic analyses of recently isolated influenza viruses, epidemiologic data, and post-vaccination serologic studies in humans, the Food and Drug Administration's Vaccines and Related Biological Products Advisory Committee (VRBPAC) recommended that the 2004–05 trivalent influenza vaccine for the United States contain A/New Caledonia/20/99-like (H1N1), A/Fujian/411/2002-like (H3N2), and B/Shanghai/361/2002-like viruses. Because of the growth properties of the A/Wyoming/3/2003 and B/Jiangsu/10/2003 viruses, US vaccine manufacturers are using these antigenically equivalent strains in the vaccine as the H3N2 and B components, respectively. The A/New Caledonia/20/99 virus will be retained as the H1N1 component of the vaccine.

2005 Season (Southern Hemisphere)

The composition of influenza virus vaccines for use in the 2005 Southern Hemisphere influenza season recommended by the World Health Organisation was:

- an A/New Caledonia/20/99(H1N1)-like virus;
- an A/Wellington/1/2004(H3N2)-like virus;
- a B/Shanghai/361/2002-like virus (B/Shanghai/361/2002, B/Jilin/20/2003 and B/Jiangsu/10/2003 were used at the time).

2005-2006 Season (Northern Hemisphere)

The vaccines produced for the 2005-2006 season use:

- an A/New Caledonia/20/1999-like(H1N1);
- an A/California/7/2004-like(H3N2) (or the antigenically equivalent strain A/New York/55/2004);
- a B/Jiangsu/10/2003-like viruses.

In people in the United States, overall flu and pneumonia deaths were below those of a typical flu season with 84 per cent Influenzavirus A and the rest Influenzavirus B. Of the patients who had Type A viruses, 80 per cent had viruses identical or similar to the A bugs in the vaccine. 70 per cent of the people testing positive for a B virus had Type B Victoria, a version not found in the vaccine.

> "During the 2005–06 season, influenza A (H3N2) viruses predominated overall, but late in the season influenza B viruses were more frequently isolated than influenza A viruses. Influenza A (H1N1) viruses circulated at low levels throughout the season. Nationally, activity was low from October through early-January, increased during February, and peaked in early-March. Peak activity was less intense, but activity remained elevated for a longer period of time this season compared to the previous three seasons. The longer period of elevated activity may be due in part to regional differences in the timing of peak activity and intensity of influenza B activity later in the season."

2006 Season (Southern Hemisphere)

The composition of influenza virus vaccines for use in the 2006 Southern Hemisphere influenza season recommended by the World Health Organisation was:

- an A/New Caledonia/20/99(H1N1)-like virus;
- an A/California/7/2004(H3N2)-like virus (A/New York/55/2004 was used at the time);
- a B/Malaysia/2506/2004-like virus.

2006-2007 Season (Northern Hemisphere)

The 2006–2007 influenza vaccine composition recommended by the World Health Organisation on February 15, 2006 and the US FDA's Vaccines and Related Biological Products Advisory Committee (VRBPAC) on February 17, 2006 use:

- an A/New Caledonia/20/99 (H1N1)-like virus;
- an A/Wisconsin/67/2005 (H3N2)-like virus (A/Wisconsin/67/2005 and A/Hiroshima/52/2005 strains);
- a B/Malaysia/2506/2004-like virus from B/Malaysia/2506/2004 and B/Ohio/1/2005 strains which are of B/Victoria/2/87 lineage.

2007 Season (Southern Hemisphere)

The composition of influenza virus vaccines for use in the 2007 Southern Hemisphere influenza season recommended by the World Health Organisation on September 20, 2006 was:

- an A/New Caledonia/20/99(H1N1)-like virus,
- an A/Wisconsin/67/2005(H3N2)-like virus (A/Wisconsin/67/2005 and A/Hiroshima/52/2005 were used at the time),
- a B/Malaysia/2506/2004-like virus

2007–2008 Season (Northern Hemisphere)

The composition of influenza virus vaccines for use in the 2007–2008 Northern Hemisphere influenza season recommended by the World Health Organisation on February 14, 2007 was:

- an A/Solomon Islands/3/2006 (H1N1)-like virus;
- an A/Wisconsin/67/2005 (H3N2)-like virus (A/Wisconsin/67/2005 (H3N2) and A/Hiroshima/52/2005 were used at the time);
- a B/Malaysia/2506/2004-like virus

In the US, the CDC reported in Feb. 2008 that the H1N1 component was a good match (96%) to the infections occurring. But 87 per cent of the H3N2 are A/Brisbane/10/2007-like viruses, which are a recent antigenic variant of the vaccine strain, A/Wisconsin. And 93 per cent of the B viruses are in a B/Yamagata lineage that is relatively distinct from the vaccine strain B/Victoria lineage. Only one of the three components was a good match; A/Wisconsin is moderately protective against the drifted A/Brisbane strain. 4.5 per cent of those viruses tested are resistant to Oseltamivir, or Tamiflu—a significant increase over previous years.

This vaccine has been described as 40 per cent effective compared to other years that have been 85-95 per cent effective.

2008 Season (Southern Hemisphere)

The composition of virus vaccines for use in the 2008 Southern Hemisphere influenza season recommended by the World Health Organisation on September 17-19, 2007 was:

- an A/Solomon Islands/3/2006 (H1N1)-like virus;
- an A/Brisbane/10/2007 (H3N2)-like virus;
- a B/Florida/4/2006-like virus.

2008-2009 Season (Northern Hemisphere)

The composition of virus vaccines for use in the 2008-2009 Northern Hemisphere influenza season recommended by the World Health Organisation on February 14, 2008 was:

- an A/Brisbane/59/2007 (H1N1)-like virus;
- an A/Brisbane/10/2007 (H3N2)-like virus;
- a B/Florida/4/2006-like virus (B/Florida/4/2006 and B/Brisbane/3/2007 (a B/Florida/4/2006-like virus) were used at the time).

As of May 30, 2009: "CDC has antigenically characterised 1,567 seasonal human influenza viruses [947 influenza A (H1), 162 influenza A (H3) and 458 influenza B viruses] collected by US laboratories since October 1, 2008, and 84 novel influenza A (H1N1) viruses. All 947 influenza seasonal A (H1) viruses are related to the influenza A (H1N1) component of the 2008-09 influenza vaccine (A/Brisbane/59/2007). All 162 influenza A (H3N2) viruses are related to the A (H3N2) vaccine component (A/Brisbane/10/2007). All 84 novel influenza A (H1N1) viruses are related to the A/California/07/2009 (H1N1) reference virus selected by WHO as a potential candidate for novel influenza A (H1N1) vaccine. Influenza B viruses currently circulating can be divided into two distinct lineages represented by the B/Yamagata/16/88 and B/Victoria/02/87 viruses. Sixty-one influenza B viruses tested belong to the B/Yamagata lineage and are related to the vaccine strain (B/Florida/04/2006). The remaining 397 viruses belong to the B/Victoria lineage and are not related to the vaccine strain."

2009 Season (Southern Hemisphere)

The composition of virus vaccines for use in the 2009 Southern Hemisphere influenza season recommended by the World Health Organisation on September 17-19, 2008 was:

- an A/Brisbane/59/2007 (H1N1)-like virus;
- an A/Brisbane/10/2007 (H3N2)-like virus;
- a B/Florida/4/2006-like virus

2009-2010 Season (Northern Hemisphere)

The composition of virus vaccines for use in the 2009-2010 Northern Hemisphere influenza season recommended by the World Health Organisation on February 12, 2009 was:

- an A/Brisbane/59/2007 (H1N1)-like virus;
- an A/Brisbane/10/2007 (H3N2)-like virus;
- a B/Brisbane/60/2008-like virus.

Since the A/Brisbane/59/2007 (H1N1)-like virus used in the vaccine is a seasonal strain of influenza, it cannot create immunity to the new, non-seasonal strain of influenza A virus subtype H1N1 responsible for the 2009 swine flu outbreak.

Flu Vaccine for Non-humans

"Vaccination in the veterinary world pursues four goals: (i) protection from clinical disease, (ii) protection from infection with virulent virus, (iii) protection from virus excretion, and (iv) serological differentiation of infected from vaccinated animals (so-called DIVA principle). In the field of influenza vaccination, neither commercially available nor experimentally tested vaccines have been shown so far to fulfil all of these requirements."

Horses: Horses with horse flu can run a fever, have a dry hacking cough, have a runny nose, and become depressed and reluctant to eat or drink for several days but usually recover in two to three weeks. "Vaccination schedules generally require a primary course of 2 doses, 3–6 weeks apart, followed by boosters at 6–12 month intervals. It is generally recognised that in many cases such schedules may not maintain protective levels of antibody and more frequent administration is advised in high-risk situations."

It is a common requirement at shows in the United Kingdom that horses are vaccinated against equine flu and a vaccination card must be produced; the FEI requires vaccination every six months.

Poultry: Poultry vaccines for bird flu are made on the cheap and are not filtered and purified like human vaccines to remove bits of bacteria or other viruses. They usually contain whole virus, not just hemagglutinin as in most human flu vaccines. Purification to standards needed for humans is far more expensive than the original creation of the unpurified vaccine from eggs.

There is no market for veterinary vaccines that are that expensive. Another difference between human and poultry vaccines is that poultry vaccines are adjuvated with mineral oil, which induces a strong immune reaction but can cause inflammation and abscesses. "Chicken vaccinators who have accidentally jabbed themselves have developed painful swollen fingers or even lost thumbs, doctors said. Effectiveness may also be limited.

Chicken vaccines are often only vaguely similar to circulating flu strains — some contain an H5N2 strain isolated in Mexico years ago. 'With a chicken, if you use a vaccine that's only 85 per cent related, you'll get protection,' Dr. Cardona said. 'In humans, you can get a single point mutation, and a vaccine that's 99.99 per cent related won't protect you.' And they are weaker [than human vaccines]. 'Chickens are smaller and you only need to protect them for six weeks, because that's how long they live till you eat them,' said Dr. John J. Treanor, a vaccine expert at the University of Rochester.

Human seasonal flu vaccines contain about 45 micrograms of antigen, while an experimental A(H5N1) vaccine contains 180. Chicken vaccines may contain less than 1 microgram. 'You have to be careful about extrapolating data from poultry to humans,' warned Dr. David E. Swayne, director of the agriculture department's Southeast Poultry Research Laboratory. 'Birds are more closely related to dinosaurs.'"

Researchers, led by Nicholas Savill of the University of Edinburgh in Scotland, used mathematical models to simulate the spread of H5N1 and concluded that "at least 95 per cent of birds need to be protected to prevent the virus spreading silently. In practice, it is difficult to protect more than 90 per cent of a flock; protection levels achieved by a vaccine are usually much lower than this."

Pigs: Swine influenza virus (SIV) vaccines are extensively used in the swine industry in Europe and North America. Most swine flu vaccine manufacturers include an H1N1 and an H3N2 SIV strains.

Swine influenza has become a greater problem in recent decades. Evolution of the virus has resulted in inconsistent responses to traditional vaccines. Standard commercial swine flu vaccines are effective in controlling the problem when the virus strains match enough to have significant cross-protection and custom (autogenous) vaccines made from the specific viruses isolated are created and used in the more difficult cases.

SIV vaccine manufacture Novartis paints this picture: "A strain of swine influenza virus (SIV) called H3N2, first identified in the US in 1998, has brought exasperating production losses to swine producers. Abortion storms are a common sign. Sows go off feed for two or three days and run a fever up to 106°F. Mortality in a naive herd can run as high as 15 per cent."

Dogs: In 2004, Influenzavirus A subtype H3N8 wa discovered to cause canine influenza. Because of the lack c previous exposure to this virus, dogs have no natural immunit to this virus.

There is no vaccine available at this time, but there ha been investigation of a canarypox-vectored vaccine for equin influenza virus for use in dogs.

8

Influenza Pandemic

An influenza pandemic is an epidemic of an influenza virus that spreads on a worldwide scale and infects a large proportion of the human population. In contrast to the regular seasonal epidemics of influenza, these pandemics occur irregularly, with the 1918 Spanish flu the most serious pandemic in recent history. Pandemics can cause high levels of mortality, with the Spanish influenza estimated as being responsible for the deaths of over 50 million people. There have been about three influenza pandemics in each century for the last 300 years. The most recent ones were the Asian Flu in 1957 and the Hong Kong Flu in 1968.

Influenza pandemics occur when a new strain of the influenza virus is transmitted to humans from another animal species. Species that are thought to be important in the emergence of new human strains are pigs, chickens and ducks. These novel strains are unaffected by any immunity people may have to older strains of human influenza and can therefore spread extremely rapidly and infect very large numbers of people. Influenza A viruses can occasionally be transmitted from wild birds to other species causing outbreaks in domestic poultry and may give rise to human influenza pandemics.

The World Health Organisation (WHO) warns that there is a substantial risk of an influenza pandemic within the next few years. One of the strongest candidates is a highly pathogenic variation of the H5N1 subtype of Influenza A virus. As of 2006, pre-pandemic influenza vaccines are being developed against the most likely suspects which include H5N1, H7N1, and H9N2. Certain scholars and senior policy advisors argue that pandemic influenza represents a substantive threat to the international economy, to national security, and a challenge to international governance.

There is current concern that the spread of a new strain of H1N1 influenza, also known as "swine flu", might develop into a pandemic. This concern about the 2009 swine flu outbreak was first raised in April 2009 by the CDC and World Health Organisation.

Influenza: Influenza, commonly known as flu, is an infectious disease of birds and mammals caused by an RNA virus of the family Orthomyxoviridae (the influenza viruses). In humans, common symptoms of influenza infection are fever, sore throat, muscle pains, severe headache, coughing, and weakness and fatigue. In more serious cases, influenza causes pneumonia, which can be fatal, particularly in young children and the elderly. Sometimes confused with the common cold, influenza is a much more severe disease and is caused by a different type of virus. Although nausea and vomiting can be produced, especially in children, these symptoms are more characteristic of the unrelated gastroenteritis, which is sometimes called "stomach flu" or "24-hour flu."

Flu spreads around the world in seasonal epidemics, killing millions of people in pandemic years and hundreds of thousands in non-pandemic years. Three influenza pandemics occurred in the 20th century and killed tens of millions of people, with each of these pandemics being caused by the appearance of a new strain of the virus in humans. Often, these new strains result from the spread of an existing flu virus to humans from other animal species. Since it first killed humans in Asia in the 1990s, a deadly avian strain of H5N1 has posed the greatest risk for a new influenza pandemic; however, this virus has not mutated to spread easily between people.

Vaccinations against influenza are most commonly given to high-risk humans in industrialised countries and to farmed poultry. The most common human vaccine is the trivalent influenza vaccine that contains purified and inactivated material from three viral strains.

Typically this vaccine includes material from two influenza A virus subtypes and one influenza B virus strain. A vaccine formulated for one year may be ineffective in the following year, since the influenza virus changes rapidly over time and different strains become dominant. Antiviral drugs can be used to treat influenza, with neuraminidase inhibitors being particularly effective.

Nature of a Flu Pandemic

Some pandemics are relatively minor such as the one in 1957 called "Asian flu" (1-4 million dead, depending on source). Others have a higher Pandemic Severity Index whose severity warrants more comprehensive social isolation measures.

The 1918 pandemic killed tens of millions and sickened hundreds of millions; the loss of this many people in the population caused upheaval and psychological damage to many people. There are not enough doctors, hospital rooms, or medical supplies for the living due to their contracting the disease and dead bodies often lie unburied as few people are available to deal with them. There is great social disruption and a sense of fear and efforts to deal with the pandemic always leave a great deal to be desired due to selfishness, lack of trust, illegal behaviour, and ignorance. For example in the 1918 pandemic: "This horrific disconnect between reassurances and reality destroyed the credibility of those in authority. People felt they had no one to turn to, no one to rely on, no one to trust."

A letter from a physician at one US Army camp in the 1918 pandemic said:

> It is only a matter of a few hours then until death comes. It is horrible. One can stand it to see one,

> two or twenty men die, but to see these poor devils dropping like flies. We have been averaging about 100 deaths per day. Pneumonia means in about all cases death. We have lost an outrageous number of nurses and doctors It takes special trains to carry away the dead. For several days there were no coffins and the bodies piled up something fierce.

Wave Nature: Flu pandemics typically come in waves. The 1889–1890 and 1918–1919 flu pandemics each came in three or four waves of increasing lethality. But within a wave, mortality was greater at the beginning of the wave.

Variable Mortality: Mortality varies widely in a pandemic. In the 1918 pandemic:

In US Army camps where reasonably reliable statistics were kept, case mortality often exceeded 5 per cent, and in some circumstances exceeded 10 per cent. In the British Army in India, case mortality for white troops was 9.6 per cent, for Indian troops 21.9 per cent. In isolated human populations, the virus killed at even higher rates. In the Fiji islands, it killed 14 per cent of the entire population in 16 days. In Labrador and Alaska, it killed at least one-third of the entire native population.

Notable Influenza Pandemics

Latest Flu Pandemics

Name of pandemic	*Date*	*Deaths*	*Subtype involved*
Asiatic (Russian) Flu	1889-90	1 million	possibly H2N2
Spanish Flu	1918-20	40 million	H1N1
Asian Flu	1957-58	1 to 1.5 million	H2N2
Hong Kong Flu	1968-69	0.75 to 1 million	H3N2

Spanish Flu (1918-1920)

The 1918 flu pandemic, commonly referred to as the Spanish flu, was a category 5 influenza pandemic caused by an unusually severe and deadly Influenza A virus strain of subtype H1N1.

The Spanish flu pandemic lasted from 1918 to 1919, although Price-Smith's data suggest it may have begun in Austria in the Spring of 1917. Older estimates say it killed 40–50 million people while current estimates say 50 million to 100 million people worldwide were killed. This pandemic has been described as "the greatest medical holocaust in history" and may have killed as many people as the Black Death, although the Black Death is estimated to have killed over a fifth of the world's population at the time, a significantly higher proportion.

Asian Flu (1957-1958)

The "Asian Flu" was a category 2 flu pandemic outbreak of avian influenza that originated in China in early-1956 lasting until 1958. It originated from mutation in wild ducks combining with a pre-existing human strain. The virus was first identified in Guizhou. It spread to Singapore in February 1957, reached Hong Kong by April, and US by June. Death toll in the US was approximately 69,800. The elderly were particularly vulnerable. Estimates of worldwide deaths vary widely depending on source, ranging from 1 million to 4 million.

Strategies to Prevent a Flu Pandemic

This section contains strategies to prevent a flu pandemic by a Council on Foreign Relations panel consisting of:

- James F. Hoge, who is Peter G. Peterson chair, editor, Foreign Affairs;
- Nancy E. Roman, who is vice president and director, Washington Programme, Council on Foreign Relations;
- Rita Colwell, who is chair, Royal Institution World Science Assembly's Pandemic Preparedness Project;
- Anthony Fauci, who is director of the National Institute of Allergy and Infectious Diseases at the National Institute of Health;
- Laurie Garrett, who is the senior fellow for global health, Council on Foreign Relations;

- Michael Osterholm, who is director of the Centre for Infectious Disease Research and Policy, University of Minnesota; also, associate director, National Centre for Food Protection and Defence, Department of Homeland Defence; also a professor at the University of Minnesota School of Public Health.

If influenza remains an animal problem with limited human-to-human transmission it is not a pandemic, though it continues to pose a risk. To prevent the situation from progressing to a pandemic, the following short-term strategies have been put forward:

- Culling and vaccinating livestock;
- Vaccinating poultry workers against common flu;
- Limiting travel in areas where the virus is found.

The rationale for vaccinating poultry workers against common flu is that it reduces the probability of common influenza virus recombining with avian H5N1 virus to form a pandemic strain. Longer term strategies proposed for regions where highly pathogenic H5N1 is endemic in wild birds have included:

- changing local farming practices to increase farm hygiene and reduce contact between livestock and wild birds;
- altering farming practices in regions where animals live in close, often unsanitary quarters with people, and changing the practices of open-air "wet markets" where birds are kept for live sale and slaughtered onsite. A challenge to implementing these measures is widespread poverty, frequently in rural areas, coupled with a reliance upon raising fowl for purposes of subsistence farming or income without measures to prevent propagation of the disease;
- changing local shopping practices from purchase of live fowl to purchase of slaughtered, pre-packaged fowl;
- improving veterinary vaccine availability and cost.

Anti-viral Drugs

Many nations, as well as the World Health Organisation, are working to stockpile antiviral drugs in preparation for a possible pandemic. Oseltamivir (trade name Tamiflu) is the most commonly sought drug, since it is available in pill form. Zanamivir (trade name Relenza) is also considered for use, but it must be inhaled. Other antiviral drugs are less likely to be effective against pandemic influenza.

Both Tamiflu and Relenza are in short supply, and production capabilities are limited in the medium term. Some doctors say that co-administration of Tamiflu with probenecid could double supplies.

There also is the potential of viruses to evolve drug resistance. Some H5N1-infected persons treated with oseltamivir have developed resistant strains of that virus.

Tamiflu was originally discovered by Gilead Sciences and licensed to Roche for late-phase development and marketing.

Public Response:

- *Social Distance:* By travelling less, working from home or closing schools there is less opportunity for the virus to spread.
- *Respiratory Hygiene:* Populations should be repeatedly informed of the need for "respiratory hygiene" (covering mouth when coughing or sneezing, careful disposal of soiled tissues or other materials).
- *Masks:* No mask can provide a perfect barrier but products that meet or exceed the NIOSH N95 standard recommended by the World Health Organisation are thought to provide good protection. WHO recommends that health-care workers wear N95 masks and that patients wear surgical masks (which may prevent respiratory secretions from becoming airborne). Any mask may be useful to remind the wearer not to touch the face. This can reduce infection due to contact with contaminated surfaces, especially in crowded public

places where coughing or sneezing people have no way of washing their hands. The mask itself can become contaminated and must be handled as medical waste when removed.

- *Hygiene:* Frequent handwashing, especially when there has been contact with other people or with potentially contaminated surfaces can be very helpful. Alcohol-based hand sanitisers also kill both bacteria and viruses.
- *Risk Communication:* To encourage the public to comply with strategies to reduce the spread of disease, "communications regarding possible community interventions [such as requiring sick people to stay home from work, closing schools] for pandemic influenza that flow from the federal government to communities and from community leaders to the public not overstate the level of confidence or certainty in the effectiveness of these measures."

The Institute of Medicine has published a number of reports and summaries of workshops on public policy issues related to influenza pandemics. They are collected in Pandemic Influenza: A Guide to Recent Institute of Medicine Studies and Workshops.

Phases: The World Health Organisation (WHO) has developed a global influenza preparedness plan, which defines the stages of a pandemic, outlines WHO's role and makes recommendations for national measures before and during a pandemic.

In the 2009 revision of the phase descriptions, WHO has retained the use of a six-phased approach for easy incorporation of new recommendations and approaches into existing national preparedness and response plans. The grouping and description of pandemic phases have been revised to make them easier to understand, more precise, and based upon observable phenomena. Phases 1–3 correlate with preparedness, including capacity development and response planning activities, while

Phases 4–6 clearly signal the need for response and mitigation efforts. Furthermore, periods after the first pandemic wave are elaborated to facilitate post-pandemic recovery activities.

The phases are defined below.

In nature, influenza viruses circulate continuously among animals, especially birds. Even though such viruses might theoretically develop into pandemic viruses, in Phase 1 no viruses circulating among animals have been reported to cause infections in humans.

In Phase 2 an animal influenza virus circulating among domesticated or wild animals is known to have caused infection in humans, and is therefore considered a potential pandemic threat.

In Phase 3, an animal or human-animal influenza reassortant virus has caused sporadic cases or small clusters of disease in people, but has not resulted in human-to-human transmission sufficient to sustain community-level outbreaks. Limited human-to-human transmission may occur under some circumstances, for example, when there is close contact between an infected person and an unprotected caregiver. However, limited transmission under such restricted circumstances does not indicate that the virus has gained the level of transmissibility among humans necessary to cause a pandemic.

Phase 4 is characterised by verified human-to-human transmission of an animal or human-animal influenza reassortant virus able to cause "community-level outbreaks." The ability to cause sustained disease outbreaks in a community marks a significant upwards shift in the risk for a pandemic. Any country that suspects or has verified such an event should urgently consult with WHO so that the situation can be jointly assessed and a decision made by the affected country if implementation of a rapid pandemic containment operation is warranted. Phase 4 indicates a significant increase in risk of a pandemic but does not necessarily mean that a pandemic is a forgone conclusion.

Phase 5 is characterised by human-to-human spread of the virus into at least two countries in one WHO region. While most countries will not be affected at this stage, the declaration of Phase 5 is a strong signal that a pandemic is imminent and that the time to finalise the organisation, communication, and implementation of the planned mitigation measures is short.

Phase 6, the pandemic phase, is characterised by community level outbreaks in at least one other country in a different WHO region in addition to the criteria defined in Phase 5. Designation of this phase will indicate that a global pandemic is under way.

During the post-peak period, pandemic disease levels in most countries with adequate surveillance will have dropped below peak observed levels. The post-peak period signifies that pandemic activity appears to be decreasing; however, it is uncertain if additional waves will occur and countries will need to be prepared for a second wave.

Previous pandemics have been characterised by waves of activity spread over months. Once the level of disease activity drops, a critical communications task will be to balance this information with the possibility of another wave. Pandemic waves can be separated by months and an immediate "at-ease" signal may be premature.

In the post-pandemic period, influenza disease activity will have returned to levels normally seen for seasonal influenza. It is expected that the pandemic virus will behave as a seasonal influenza A virus. At this stage, it is important to maintain surveillance and update pandemic preparedness and response plans accordingly. An intensive phase of recovery and evaluation may be required.

Preparations for a Potential Influenza Pandemic

According to *The New York Times* as of March 2006, "governments worldwide have spent billions planning for a potential influenza pandemic: buying medicines, running disaster drills, [and] developing strategies for tighter border controls" due to the H5N1 threat.

The United States is collaborating closely with eight international organisations, including the World Health Organisation (WHO), the Food and Agriculture Organisation of the United Nations (FAO), the World Organisation for Animal Health (OIE), and 88 foreign governments to address the situation through planning, greater monitoring, and full transparency in reporting and investigating avian influenza occurrences. The United States and these international partners have led global efforts to encourage countries to heighten surveillance for outbreaks in poultry and significant numbers of deaths in migratory birds and to rapidly introduce containment measures. The US Agency for International Development (USAID) and the US Departments of State, Health and Human Services (HHS), and Agriculture (USDA) are coordinating future international response measures on behalf of the White House with departments and agencies across the federal government.

Together steps are being taken to "minimise the risk of further spread in animal populations", "reduce the risk of human infections", and "further support pandemic planning and preparedness".

Ongoing detailed mutually coordinated onsite surveillance and analysis of human and animal H5N1 avian flu outbreaks are being conducted and reported by the USGS National Wildlife Health Centre, the Centres for Disease Control and Prevention, the World Health Organisation, the European Commission, the National Influenza Centres, and others.

Canada: The Public Health Agency of Canada follows the WHO's categories, but has expanded them. The Avian Flu scare of 2006 prompted The Canadian Public Health Agency to release an updated Pandemic Influenza Plan for Health Officials. This document was created to address the growing concern over the hazards faced by public health officials when exposed to sick or dying patients.

Some Canadian health officials contend that the known nature of influenza outbreaks are not as hazardous to public health as unknown respiratory disorders like SARS.

China: In 1982, Kennedy F. Shortridge and Charles Stuart-Harris proposed that China, particularly southern China, is a centre for the emergence of pandemic influenza viruses. This hypothesis was based on three observations:

1. The occurrence of a large number of viruses in domestic poultry, notably ducks, in the region.
2. The dense populations and proximity of humans, poultry and pigs in villages and farms there.
3. The historical records associating China with epidemics and pandemics and, in the last century, the association of southern China with the emergence of the 1957 Asian and 1968 Hong Kong pandemic strains and the re-emergence of the 1977 H1N1 virus. These records have been reinforced by the 1997 H5N1 incident that is considered by some to have been an incipient pandemic and a pandemic averted by the slaughter of poultry across Hong Kong SAR in late-1997.

United Nations: In September 2005, David Nabarro, a lead UN health official warned that a bird flu outbreak could happen anytime and had the potential to kill 5–150 million people.

United States: "Efforts by the federal government to prepare for pandemic influenza at the national level include a $100 million DHHS initiative in 2003 to build US vaccine production. Several agencies within Department of Health and Human Services (DHHS) — including the Office of the Secretary, the Food and Drug Administration (FDA), CDC, and the National Institute of Allergy and Infectious Diseases (NIAID) — are in the process of working with vaccine manufacturers to facilitate production of pilot vaccine lots for both H5N1 and H9N2 strains as well as contracting for the manufacturing of 2 million doses of an H5N1 vaccine. This H5N1 vaccine production will provide a critical pilot test of the pandemic vaccine system; it will also be used for clinical trials to evaluate dose and immunogenicity and can provide initial vaccine for early use in the event of an emerging pandemic."

On August 26, 2004, Secretary of Health and Human Services, Tommy Thompson released a draft Pandemic Influenza Response and Preparedness Plan, which outlined a coordinated national strategy to prepare for and respond to an influenza pandemic. Public comments were accepted for 60 days.

In a speech before the United Nations General Assembly on September 14, 2005, President George W. Bush announced the creation of the International Partnership on Avian and Pandemic Influenza. The Partnership brings together nations and international organisations to improve global readiness by:

- elevating the issue on national agendas;
- coordinating efforts among donor and affected nations;
- mobilising and leveraging resources;
- increasing transparency in disease reporting and surveillance; and
- building capacity to identify, contain and respond to a pandemic influenza.

On October 5, 2005, Democratic Senators Harry Reid, Evan Bayh, Dick Durbin, Ted Kennedy, Barack Obama, and Tom Harkin introduced the Pandemic Preparedness and Response Act as a proposal to deal with a possible outbreak.

On October 27, 2005, the Department of Health and Human Services awarded a $62.5 million contract to Chiron Corporation to manufacture an avian influenza vaccine designed to protect against the H5N1 influenza virus strain. This followed a previous awarded $100 million contract to sanofi Pasteur, the vaccines business of the sanofi-aventis Group, for avian flu vaccine.

In October 2005, President Bush urged bird flu vaccine manufacturers to increase their production.

On November 1, 2005 President Bush unveiled the National Strategy To Safeguard Against The Danger of Pandemic Influenza. He also submitted a request to Congress for $7.1 billion to begin implementing the plan. The request includes $251 million to detect and contain outbreaks before they spread around the world; $2.8 billion to accelerate development of cell-culture technology; $800 million for development of new treatments and vaccines; $1.519 billion for the Departments of Health and Human Services (HHS) and Defence to purchase influenza vaccines; $1.029 billion to stockpile antiviral medications; and $644 million to ensure that all levels of government are prepared to respond to a pandemic outbreak.

On 6 March 2006, Mike Leavitt, Secretary of Health and Human Services, said US health agencies are continuing to develop vaccine alternatives that will protect against the evolving avian influenza virus.

The US government, bracing for the possibility that migrating birds could carry a deadly strain of bird flu to North America, plans to test nearly eight times as many wild birds starting in April 2006 as have been tested in the past decade.

On 8 March 2006, Dr. David Nabarro, senior UN coordinator for avian and human influenza, said that given the flight patterns of wild birds that have been spreading avian influenza (bird flu) from Asia to Europe and Africa, birds infected with the H5N1 virus could reach the Americas within the next six to 12 months.

"Jul. 5, 2006 (CIDRAP News) – In an update on pandemic influenza preparedness efforts, the federal government said last week it had stockpiled enough vaccine against H5N1 avian influenza virus to inoculate about 4 million people and enough antiviral medication to treat about 6.3 million."

World Health Organisation Plan

The World Health Organisation (WHO) believes that the world is currently closer to another influenza pandemic than it has been any time since 1968, when the last of the 20th century's three pandemics swept the globe and has developed a global influenza preparedness plan outlining the role of the WHO and recommendations for national measures before and during pandemics.

9

Effect on Human Society

Influenza has had a huge effect on human society, especially the financial, political, social, and personal responses to both actual and predicted deaths in birds, humans, and other animals.

Billions of US dollars are being raised and spent to research and prepare for a potential avian influenza pandemic. Over ten billion dollars have been spent and over two hundred million birds killed to try to contain the virus.

People have reacted by buying less chicken causing poultry sales and prices to fall. Many individuals have stockpiled supplies for a possible flu pandemic. One of the best known experts on H5N1, Dr. Robert Webster, told ABC News he had a three month supply of food and water in his house as he prepared for what he considered a reasonably likely occurrence of a major pandemic.

International health officials and other experts have pointed out that many unknown questions still hover around the disease

Dr. David Nabarro, Chief Avian Flu Coordinator for the United Nations, and former Chief of Crisis Response for the World Health Organisation has described himself as "quite scared" about H5N1's potential impact on humans. Nabarro has been accused of being alarmist before and on his first day in his role for the United Nations he proclaimed the avian flu could kill 150 million people. In an interview with the

International Herald Tribune, Nabarro compares avian flu to AIDS in Africa, warning that underestimations led to inappropriate focus for research and intervention.

Affecting Virus

Influenza A Virus Subtype H5N2

H5N2 and Birds: Low pathogenic avian influenza H5N2 virus in poultry later gained accentuated virulence in the United States and Mexico. A highly pathogenic strain of H5N2 caused flu outbreaks with significant spread to numerous farms, resulting in great economic losses in 1983 in Pennsylvania, USA in chickens and turkeys, in 1994 in Mexico in chickens and a minor outbreak in 1997 in Italy in chickens.

In Korea, ducks have been destroyed at the farm since quarantine officials detected the suspected low pathogenic H5N2 strain of avian influenza on December 1, 2004.

In Japan, H5N2 virus was isolated or an anti-H5 antibody was identified from chickens in 40 chicken farms in Ibaraki Prefecture and in one chicken farm in Saitama Prefecture from June through December 2005. The strain was named as A/ chicken /Ibaraki/1/2005(H5N2). About 5.7 million birds were destroyed in Ibaraki following the H5N2 outbreaks.

It was reported on November 12, 2005 that "One of 2 birds found infected with bird flu in Kuwait has the H5N1 strain of the virus, authorities said. The infected bird was a migrating flamingo found on a Kuwait beach. The other was an imported falcon found to have the milder H5N2 variant."

In China, inactivated H5N2 has been used as a vaccine for H5N1.

In 2006, an H5N2 outbreak on a single farm in South Africa resulted in the destruction of all its sixty ostriches. The strain was similar to the one that caused outbreaks in South Africa 2004/2005.

In 2007, a low-pathogenic strain of H5N2 was found in samples collected from 25,000 turkeys in Pendleton County,

West Virginia in a routine testing prior to their slaughter. The birds showed no sign of illness or mortality. Measures were taken to prevent the virus from mutating and spreading.

In late-2007 (December 21), an H5N2 outbreak was found in the Dominican Republic, in a Suburb of Higuey City, on the eastern side of the island. 15 roosters and 2 hens where eliminated even though they had no visible sign of infection.

In May and June 2008, there were three outbreaks of low-pathogenic H5N2 avian flu in birds at three locations in the central, northern, and southern parts of Haiti. "The outbreaks began on May 20 and appeared to be ongoing", as of June 17, 2008.

In Taiwan, outbreaks of H5N2 have been confirmed in December 2008.

H5N2 and Humans: Japan's Health Ministry said Jan., 2006 that poultry farm workers in Ibaraki prefecture may have been exposed to H5N2 (which was not previously known to infect humans) in 2005. Data were collected from 257 workers at 35 chicken farms by Ibaraki prefectural government. Using a Wilcoxon signed-rank test, it was determined that the H5N2 antibody titers of the second samples of paired sera were significantly higher than those of the first samples. The H5N2 antibody titers of paired sera of 13 subjects increased fourfold or more. The results suggest that this may have been the first avian influenza H5N2 infection from poultry to affect humans.

Influenza A Virus Subtype H5N3

H5N3 is a subtype of the species Influenza A virus (sometimes called bird flu virus).

H5N3 was identified in Quebec in August 2005 and in Sweden in October 2005.

2009: H5N3 virus was identified at a La Garnache farm in France in late-January. 90 birds were found dead between 29 January 2009 and 31 January 2009. The remaining stock of 4932 birds was destroyed on 1 February 2009.

Influenza A Virus Subtype H5N8

H5N8 is a subtype of the species Influenza A virus (sometimes called bird flu virus).

A highly pathogenic strain of it called A/Turkey/Ireland/1378/83 caused a minor flu outbreak in 1983 in Ireland in turkeys.

Influenza A Virus Subtype H5N9

H5N9 is a subtype of the species Influenza A virus (sometimes called bird flu virus).

A highly pathogenic strain of H5N9 caused a minor flu outbreak in 1966 in Ontario, Canada in turkeys.

Influenza A Virus Subtype H7N1

H7N1 is a subtype of the species Influenza A virus (sometimes called bird flu virus).

A highly pathogenic strain of it caused a flu outbreak with significant spread to numerous farms, resulting in great economic losses in 1999 in Italy in turkeys.

Influenza A Virus Subtype H7N2

H7N2 is a subtype of the species Influenza A virus (sometimes called bird flu virus).

One person in Virginia, US in 2002 and one person in New York, US, in 2003 were found to have serologic evidence of infection from H7N2; both fully recovered.

In February 2004, an outbreak of low pathogenic avian influenza (LPAI) A (H7N2) was reported on 2 chicken farms in Delaware and in four live bird markets in New Jersey supplied by the same farms. In March 2004, surveillance samples from a flock of chickens in Maryland tested positive for LPAI H7N2. It is likely that this was the same strain.

A CDC study following the 2002 outbreaks of H7N2 in commercial poultry farms in western Virginia concluded:

An important factor contributing to rapid early spread of AI virus infection among commercial poultry farms during this outbreak was disposal of dead birds via rendering off-farm. Because of the highly infectious nature of AI virus and the devastating economic impact of outbreaks, poultry farmers should consider carcass disposal techniques that do not require off-farm movement, such as burial, composting, or incineration.

On 24 May 2007, an outbreak of H7N2 was confirmed at a poultry farm near Corwen, in Wales from tests on chickens that died from H7N2. The owners of the Conwy farm bought 15 Rhode Island Red chickens two weeks prior but all died from H7N2. The 32 other poultry at the site were slaughtered. A one kilometre exclusion zone was put in force around the property in which birds and bird products cannot be moved and bird gathering can only take place under licence. Nine people who were associated with the infected or dead poultry and reported flu-like symptoms were tested. Four tested positive for evidence of infection from H7N2 and were successfully treated for mild flu. In early-June it was discovered that the virus had spread to a poultry farm 70 miles (113 km) away near St. Helens in northwest England. All the poultry at the farm were slaughtered and a 1 km exclusion zone imposed.

A 2008 analysis of the New York 2003 case concluded that the H7N2 virus responsible could be evolving towards the same strong sugar-binding properties of the three worldwide viral pandemics in 1918, 1957 and 1968. (Human flus and bird flus differ in the molecules they are good at binding with because mammals and birds differ in the molecules on the cell surface to be bound with. Humans have very few cells with the bird sugar on its cell surface.) A study with ferrets showed that this H7N2 strain could be passed from mammal to mammal.

Influenza A Virus Subtype H7N3

H7N3 is a subtype of the species Influenza A virus (sometimes called bird flu virus).

In North America, the presence of H7N3 was confirmed at several poultry farms in British Columbia in February 2004. As of April 2004, 18 farms had been quarantined to halt the spread of the virus. Two cases of humans infected with it have been confirmed in that region. Symptoms included conjunctivitis and mild influenza-like illness. Both fully recovered.

> "The H7N3 strain was first detected in turkeys in Britain in 1963 and made one of its last known appearances in poultry in Canada in April and May 2004, according to the WHO and World Organisation for Animal Health. An outbreak of the less virulent H5N2 strain of bird flu in Taiwan in 2004 led to the culling of hundreds of thousands of fowl."

> "Taiwan found a highly pathogenic strain of avian flu, H7N3, in droppings left by a migratory bird and is carrying out tests to see whether the virus has spread to nearby poultry farms, the agriculture department said 14 November 2005."

For the first time since 1979, H7N3 was found in the UK in April 2006. It infected birds and one poultry worker (whose only symptom was conjunctivitis) in a Norfolk, England Witford Lodge Farm. "Antiviral Tamiflu was administered to poultry workers on the farm as a precautionary measure. [...] 35,000 chickens will be culled in the infected farm and a 1 kilometre exclusion zone has been placed."

In September 27, 2007 another outbreak of H7N3 was detected in a poultry operation in Saskatchewan, Canada. The Canadian Food Inspection Agency has requested the euthanisation of the flock, and the disinfection of all building, materials and equipment in contact with the birds or their droppings.

Influenza A Virus Subtype H7N4

H7N4 is a subtype of the species Influenza A virus (sometimes called bird flu virus).

A highly pathogenic strain of it caused a minor flu outbreak in 1997 in New South Wales, Australia in chicken.

Influenza A Virus Subtype H7N7

H7N7 is a subtype of Influenzavirus A, a genus of Orthomyxovirus, the viruses responsible for influenza. Highly pathogenic strains (HPAI) and low pathogenic strains (LPAI) exist. H7N7 can infect humans, birds, pigs, seals, and horses in the wild; and has infected mice in laboratory studies. This unusual zoonotic potential represents a pandemic threat.

In 2003 in the Netherlands 89 people were confirmed to have the H7N7 influenza virus infection following an outbreak in poultry on several farms. One death was recorded. Antibodies were found in over half of 500 persons tested according to the final official report by the Dutch government:

As at least 50 per cent of the people exposed to infected poultry had H7 antibodies detectable with the modified assay, it was estimated that avian influenza A/H7N7 virus infection occurred in at least 1000, and perhaps as many as 2000 people. The seroprevalence of H7 antibodies in people without contact with infected poultry, but with close household contact to an infected poultry worker, was 59 per cent. This suggests that the population at risk for avian influenza was not limited to those with direct contact to infected poultry, and that person to person transmission may have occurred on a large scale. Final analysis of Dutch avian influenza outbreaks reveals much higher levels of transmission to humans than previously thought .

In August 2006, low pathogenic (LP) H7N7 was found during routine testing at a poultry farm in Voorthuizen in the central Netherlands. As a precautionary measure, 25,000 chickens were culled from Voorthuizen and surrounding farms.

In June 2008, high pathogenic (HP) H7N7 was confirmed on a 25,000-bird laying unit at Shenington, England; probably derived from a pre-existing low pathogenic variety. "Increased mortality (2.5 per cent in one shed) and a drop in egg production had been recorded two weeks before birds started dying in large numbers on June 2, leading to the diagnosis of HP H7N7 on June 4."

Influenza A Virus Subtype H9N2

H9N2 is a subtype of the species Influenza A virus (sometimes called bird flu virus). In 1999 and 2003, an H9N2 influenza strain caused illness in three people, aged one, four and five years old, in Hong Kong. All three patients recovered. In 2007 an H9N2 influenza strain caused illness in a 9-month-old baby in Hong Kong.

H9N2 influenza viruses of domestic ducks have become established in the domestic poultry of Asia. Phylogenetic and antigenic analyses of the H9N2 viruses isolated from Hong Kong markets suggest three distinct sublineages. Among the chicken H9N2 viruses, six of the gene segments were apparently derived from an earlier chicken H9N2 virus isolated in China, whereas the PB1 and PB2 genes are closely related to those of the H5N1 viruses and a quail H9N2 virus A/quail/Hong Kong/G1/97 (Qa/HK/G1/97) suggesting that many of the 1997 chicken H9 isolates in the markets were reassortants.

The National Institute of Allergy and Infectious Diseases (NIAID), part of the National Institutes of Health (NIH), has issued a task order under an existing contract to Chiron Corporation of Emeryville, CA, for the production of an investigational vaccine based on an H9N2 strain of avian influenza virus that has infected humans and has the potential to trigger a modern-day pandemic.

Influenza A Virus Subtype H10N7

H10N7 is a subtype of the species Influenza A virus (sometimes called bird flu virus). In 2004 in Egypt H10N7 was reported for the first time in humans. It caused illness in two one-year-old infants, residents of Ismaillia, Egypt; one child's father a poultry merchant.

The first reported H10N7 outbreak in the US occurred in Minnesota on two turkey farms in 1979 and on a third in 1980. "The clinical signs ranged from severe, with a mortality rate as high as 31 per cent, to subclinical. Antigenically indistinguishable viruses were isolated from healthy mallards on a pond adjacent to the turkey farms"

Outbreak in Humans 2009

The 2009 flu outbreak is due to a new strain of subtype H1N1 not previously reported in pigs. In late-April, Margaret Chan, the World Health Organisation's director-general, declared a "public health emergency of international concern" under the rules of the WHO's new International Health Regulations when the first cases of the H1N1 virus were reported in the United States. Following the outbreak, on May 2, 2009, it was reported in pigs at a farm in Alberta, Canada, with a link to the outbreak in Mexico. The pigs are suspected to have caught this new strain of virus from a farm worker who recently returned from Mexico, then showed symptoms of an influenza-like illness. These are probable cases, pending confirmation by laboratory testing.

The new strain was initially described as apparent reassortment of at least four strains of influenza A virus subtype H1N1, including one strain endemic in humans, one endemic in birds, and two endemic in swine. Subsequent analysis suggested it was a reassortment of just two strains, both found in swine. Although initial reports identified the new strain as swine influenza (i.e., a zoonosis originating in swine), its origin is unknown. Several countries took precautionary measures to reduce the chances for a global pandemic of the disease. The Swine flu has been compared to other similar types of influenza virus in terms of mortality *"in the US it appears that for every 1000 people who get infected, about 40 people need admission to hospital and about one person dies"*.

10

Influenza Outbreak 2009

Minor outbreaks of swine influenza occurred in humans in 1976 and 1988, and in pigs in 1998 and 2007.

In the 2009 swine flu outbreak, the virus isolated from patients in the United States was found to be made up of genetic elements from four different flu viruses – North American Mexican influenza, North American avian influenza, human influenza, and swine influenza virus typically found in Asia and Europe – "an unusually mongrelised mix of genetic sequences." This new strain appears to be a result of reassortment of human influenza and swine influenza viruses, in all four different strains of subtype H1N1.

However, as the virus has not yet been isolated in animals to date and also for historical naming reasons, the World Organisation for Animal Health (OIE) suggests it be called "North-American influenza". On April 30, 2009 the World Health Organisation began referring to the outbreak as "Influenza A" instead of "swine flu"., and later began referring to it as "Influenza A(H1N1)". Several complete genome sequences for US flu cases were rapidly made available through the Global Initiative on Sharing Avian Influenza Data (GISAID). Preliminary genetic characterisation found that the hemagglutinin (HA) gene was similar to that of swine flu viruses present in US pigs since 1999, but the neuraminidase

(NA) and matrix protein (M) genes resembled versions present in European swine flu isolates. The six genes from American swine flu are themselves mixtures of swine flu, bird flu, and human flu viruses. While viruses with this genetic makeup had not previously been found to be circulating in humans or pigs, there is no formal national surveillance system to determine what viruses are circulating in pigs in the US.

Influenza Virus Subtypes

Influenza A Virus Subtype H1N1

Influenza A virus subtype H1N1, also known as A(H1N1), is a subtype of influenzavirus A and the most common cause of influenza (flu) in humans. Some strains of H1N1 are endemic in humans, including the strain(s) responsible for the 1918 flu pandemic which killed 50-100 million people worldwide. Less virulent H1N1 strains still exist in the wild today, worldwide, causing a small fraction of all influenza-like illness and a large fraction of all seasonal influenza. H1N1 strains caused roughly half of all flu infections in 2006. Other strains of H1N1 are endemic in pigs (swine influenza) and in birds (avian influenza).

In March to June of 2009, thousands of laboratory-confirmed infections and a number of deaths were caused by an outbreak of a new strain of H1N1.

Nomenclature

Influenza A virus strains are categorised according to two proteins found on the surface of the virus: hemagglutinin (H) and neuraminidase (N). All influenza A viruses contain hemagglutinin and neuraminidase, but the structure of these proteins differ from strain to strain due to rapid genetic mutation in the viral genome.

Influenza A virus strains are assigned an H number and an N number based on which forms of these two proteins the strain contains. There are 16 H and 9 N subtypes known in birds, but only H 1, 2 and 3, and N 1 and 2 are commonly found in humans.

Spanish Flu

The Spanish flu, also known as *La Gripe Espanola*, or *La Pesadilla*, was an unusually severe and deadly strain of avian influenza, a viral infectious disease, that killed some 50 million to 100 million people worldwide over about a year in 1918 and 1919. It is thought to be one of the most deadly pandemics in human history. It was caused by the H1N1 type of influenza virus.

The Spanish flu caused an unusual number of deaths because it may have caused a cytokine storm in the body. (The recent epidemic of bird flu, also an Influenza A virus, had a similar effect.) The Spanish flu virus infected lung cells, leading to overstimulation of the immune system via release of cytokines into the lung tissue. This leads to extensive leukocyte migration towards the lungs, causing destruction of lung tissue and secretion of liquid into the organ. This makes it difficult for the patient to breathe. In contrast to other pandemics, which mostly kill the old and the very young, the 1918 pandemic killed unusual numbers of young adults, which may have been due to their healthy immune systems being able to mount a very strong and damaging response to the infection.

The term "Spanish" flu was coined because Spain was at the time the only European country where the press were printing reports of the outbreak, which had killed thousands in the armies fighting the First World War. Other countries suppressed the news in order to protect morale.

Russian Flu

The more recent Russian flu was a 1977-1978 flu epidemic caused by strain *Influenza A/USSR/90/77 (H1N1)*. It infected mostly children and young adults under 23 because a similar strain was prevalent in 1947-57, causing most adults to have substantial immunity. Some have called it a flu pandemic but because it only affected the young it is not considered a true pandemic. The virus was included in the 1978-1979 influenza vaccine.

Influenza A Virus Subtype H1N2

H1N2 is a subtype of the species Influenza A virus (sometimes called bird flu virus). It is currently pandemic in both human and pig populations.

H1N1, H1N2, and H3N2 are the only known Influenza A virus subtypes currently circulating among humans.

The new A(H1N2) strain appears to have resulted from the reassortment of the genes of the currently circulating influenza A(H1N1) and A(H3N2) subtypes. The hemagglutinin protein of the A(H1N2) virus is similar to that of the currently circulating A(H1N1) viruses and the neuraminidase protein is similar to that of the current A(H3N2) viruses.

It is unknown where the A(H1N2) virus originated, but on February 6, 2002, the World Health Organisation (WHO) in Geneva and the Public Health Laboratory Service (PHLS) in the United Kingdom reported the identification influenza A(H1N2) virus from humans in the UK, Israel, and Egypt. In addition to the virus isolates reported by WHO and PHLS, the Centres for Disease Control and Prevention has identified influenza A(H1N2) virus from patient specimens collected during the 2001-2002 and 2002-2003 seasons.* Influenza A(H1N2) viruses have circulated transiently in the past. Between December 1988 and March 1989, 19 influenza A(H1N2) virus isolates were identified in 6 cities in China, but the virus did not spread further.

A(H1N2) was also identified during the 2001-2002 flu season (northern hemisphere) in Canada, the USA, Ireland, Latvia, France, Romania, Oman, India, Malaysia, and Singapore.

The H1N2 virus is not very different from the currently circulating influenza viruses. The H1 protein of the H1N2 virus is like the H1 protein of the currently circulating H1N1 viruses and the N2 protein is similar to the N2 protein in the currently circulating H3N2 viruses. The difference is that we don't commonly see the H1 and N2 proteins on the same virus.

The A(H1N2) virus is not causing a more severe illness than other influenza viruses, and no unusual increases in influenza activity have been associated with the A(H1N2) virus. Because both the hemagglutinin and neuraminidase protein on the A(H1N2) virus closely matches the hemagglutinin and neuraminidase proteins of viruses included in the current influenza vaccine, the vaccine should provide good protection against influenza A(H1N2) virus as well as protection against the currently circulating A(H1N1), A(H3N2), and B viruses.

Influenza A Virus Subtype H2N2

H2N2 is a subtype of the species Influenza A virus (sometimes called bird flu virus). H2N2 has mutated into various strains including the Asian Flu strain (now extinct in the wild), H3N2, and various strains found in birds. It is also suspected of causing a human pandemic in 1889.

Russian Flu

Some believe that the 1889-1890 Russian flu was caused by influenza A virus subtype H2N2, but the evidence is not conclusive. It is the earliest flu pandemic for which detailed records are available. In 1889 it "began in Russia and spread rapidly throughout Europe. It reached North America in December 1889 and spread to Latin America and Asia in February 1890. About 1 million people died in this pandemic."

Asian Flu

The "Asian Flu" was a category 2 flu pandemic outbreak of avian influenza that originated in China in early-1956 lasting until 1958. It originated from mutation in wild ducks combining with a pre-existing human strain. The virus was first identified in Guizhou. It spread to Singapore in February 1957, reached Hong Kong by April, and US by June. Death toll in the US was approximately 69,800. Estimates of worldwide death rate varies widely depending on source, ranging from 1 million to 4 million.

Asian Flu was of the H2N2 strain (a notation that refers to the configuration of the hemagglutinin and neuraminidase proteins in the virus) of type A influenza, and an influenza vaccine was developed in 1957 to contain its outbreak.

The Asian Flu strain later evolved via antigenic shift into H3N2 which caused a milder pandemic from 1968 to 1969.

Both the H2N2 and H3N2 pandemic strains contained avian influenza virus RNA segments. "While the pandemic human influenza viruses of 1957 (H2N2) and 1968 (H3N2) clearly arose through reassortment between human and avian viruses, the influenza virus causing the 'Spanish flu' in 1918 appears to be entirely derived from an avian source (Belshe 2005)."

Test Kits

From October 2004 to February 2005, approximately 3,700 test kits of the 1957 H2N2 virus were accidentally spread around the world from the College of American Pathologists (CAP). CAP assists laboratories in accuracy by providing unidentified samples of viruses; private contractor Meridian Bioscience in Cincinnati, US, chose the 1957 strand instead of one of the less deadly avian influenza virus subtypes. "CAP spokesman Dr. Jared Schwartz said Meridian knew what the virus was but believed it was safe. In selecting it, the company had determined that the virus was classified as a biosafety level 2 (BSL-2) agent, which meant it could legally be used in the kits. [...] Before the problem came to light, the CDC had made a recommendation that the H2N2 virus be reclassified as a BSL-3 agent, Gerberding said. She promised to speed up the reclassification. The CDC determines the classifications in collaboration with the National Institutes of Health. In BSL-3 labs, agents are handled with equipment designed to prevent any airborne contamination and resulting respiratory exposure." The 1957 H2N2 virus is considered deadly and the US government called for the vials containing the strain to be destroyed.

> "CDC officials reported on 21 April that 99 per cent of the samples had already been destroyed. News reports on 25 April said the last samples outside the United States had been destroyed at the American University of Beirut in Lebanon, after

they were found at the Beirut airport. Earlier reports said H2N2 samples were sent to 3,747 labs under CAP auspices and to about another 2,700 labs certified by other organisations. All but about 75 labs that received the CAP samples were in the United States."

"In the United States, there is no government regulation over the 1957 flu strain. In fact, federal officials at the CDC do not even know how many US laboratories keep this deadly strain in their viral libraries."

Influenza A Virus Subtype H3N1

H3N1 is a subtype of the species Influenza A virus, mostly affecting pigs.

The known subtypes of Influenza A virus that create influenza in pigs and are endemic in pigs are H1N1, H1N2, H3N1 and H3N2.

Influenza A Virus Subtype H3N2

Influenza A virus subtype H3N2 (also H3N2) is a subtype of viruses that cause influenza (flu). H3N2 viruses can infect birds and mammals. In birds, humans, and pigs, the virus has mutated into many strains. H3N2 is increasingly abundant in seasonal influenza, which kills an estimated 36,000 people in the United States each year.

2009 H1N1 Influenza Outbreak

The British Columbia Centre for Disease Control reported on 5 May 2009 that on 28 April 2009 it had isolated a new variant H3N2 virus from a person who recently visited Mexico. It has been suggested that some of the differences in the pathology of the influenza in Mexico may be due to the presence of this variant H3N2 and not H1N1.

The Backdrop

H3N8 is suspected of causing a human influenza pandemic in either 1889 or 1900. Sources differ; some say the 1889 pandemic was caused by H2N2. The experts also differ on exactly how sure we can be that either were involved.

A 1997 study found H3N8 was responsible for over one quarter of the influenza infections in wild ducks.

Other Subtypes

Influenza A Virus Subtype H3N8

H3N8 is a subtype of the species Influenza A virus that is endemic in birds, horses and dogs.

Influenza A Virus Subtype H5N1

Influenza A virus subtype H5N1, also known as "bird flu," A(H5N1) or simply H5N1, is a subtype of the Influenza A virus which can cause illness in humans and many other animal species. A bird-adapted strain of H5N1, called HPAI A(H5N1) for "highly pathogenic avian influenza virus of type A of subtype H5N1", is the causative agent of H5N1 flu, commonly known as "avian influenza" or "bird flu". It is enzootic in many bird populations, especially in South East Asia. One strain of HPAI A(H5N1) is spreading globally after first appearing in Asia. It is epizootic (an epidemic in non-humans) and panzootic (affecting animals of many species, especially over a wide area), killing tens of millions of birds and spurring the culling of hundreds of millions of others to stem its spread. Most references to "bird flu" and H5N1 in the popular media refer to this strain.

According to the FAO Avian Influenza Disease Emergency Situation Update, H5N1 pathogenicity is continuing to gradually rise in wild birds in endemic areas but the avian influenza disease situation in farmed birds is being held in check by vaccination. Eleven outbreaks of H5N1 were reported worldwide in June 2008 in five countries (China, Egypt, Indonesia, Pakistan and Vietnam) compared to 65 outbreaks in June 2006 and 55 in June 2007. The "global HPAI situation can be said to have improved markedly in the first half of 2008 [but] cases of HPAI are still underestimated and underreported in many countries because of limitations in country disease surveillance systems".

Overview

HPAI A(H5N1) is considered an avian disease, although there is some evidence of limited human-to-human transmission of the virus. A risk factor for contracting the virus is handling of infected poultry, but transmission of the virus from infected birds to humans is inefficient. Still, around 60 per cent of humans known to have been infected with the current Asian strain of HPAI A(H5N1) have died from it, and H5N1 may mutate or reassort into a strain capable of efficient human-to-human transmission.

In 2003, world-renowned virologist Robert Webster published an article titled "The world is teetering on the edge of a pandemic that could kill a large fraction of the human population" in *American Scientist*. He called for adequate resources to fight what he sees as a major world threat to possibly billions of lives.

On September 29, 2005, David Nabarro, the newly-appointed Senior United Nations System Coordinator for Avian and Human Influenza, warned the world that an outbreak of avian influenza could kill anywhere between 5 million and 150 million people. Experts have identified key events (creating new clades, infecting new species, spreading to new areas) marking the progression of an avian flu virus towards becoming pandemic, and many of those key events have occurred more rapidly than expected.

Due to the high lethality and virulence of HPAI A(H5N1), its endemic presence, its increasingly large host reservoir, and its significant ongoing mutations, the H5N1 virus is the world's largest current pandemic threat and billions of dollars are being spent researching H5N1 and preparing for a potential influenza pandemic. At least 12 companies and 17 governments are developing pre-pandemic influenza vaccines in 28 different clinical trials that, if successful, could turn a deadly pandemic infection into a non-deadly one. Full-scale production of a vaccine that could prevent any illness at all from the strain would require at least three months after the virus's emergence to begin, but it is hoped that vaccine production could increase until one billion doses were produced by one year after the initial identification of the virus.

H5N1 may cause more than one influenza pandemic as it is expected to continue mutating in birds regardless of whether humans develop herd immunity to a future pandemic strain. Influenza pandemics from its genetic offspring may include influenza A virus subtypes other than H5N1. While genetic analysis of the H5N1 virus shows that influenza pandemics from its genetic offspring can easily be far more lethal than the Spanish Flu pandemic, planning for a future influenza pandemic is based on what can be done and there is no higher Pandemic Severity Index level than a Category 5 pandemic which, roughly speaking, is any pandemic as bad as the Spanish flu or worse; and for which *all* intervention measures are to be used.

Genetics

The first known strain of HPAI A(H5N1) (called A/chicken/Scotland/59) killed two flocks of chickens in Scotland in 1959; but that strain was very different from the current highly pathogenic strain of H5N1. The dominant strain of HPAI A(H5N1) in 2004 evolved from 1999 to 2002 creating the Z genotype. It has also been called "Asian lineage HPAI A(H5N1)".

Asian lineage HPAI A(H5N1) is divided into two antigenic clades. "Clade 1 includes human and bird isolates from Vietnam, Thailand, and Cambodia and bird isolates from Laos and Malaysia. Clade 2 viruses were first identified in bird isolates from China, Indonesia, Japan, and South Korea before spreading westward to the Middle East, Europe, and Africa. The clade 2 viruses have been primarily responsible for human H5N1 infections that have occurred during late-2005 and 2006, according to WHO. Genetic analysis has identified six subclades of clade 2, three of which have a distinct geographic distribution and have been implicated in human infections:

- Subclade 1, Indonesia;
- Subclade 2, Europe, Middle East, and Africa (called EMA);
- Subclade 3, China".

A 2007 study focused on the EMA subclade has shed further light on the EMA mutations. "The 36 new isolates reported here greatly expand the amount of whole-genome sequence data available from recent avian influenza (H5N1) isolates. Before our project, GenBank contained only 5 other complete genomes from Europe for the 2004-2006 period, and it contained no whole genomes from the Middle East or northern Africa. Our analysis showed several new findings.

First, all European, Middle Eastern, and African samples fall into a clade that is distinct from other contemporary Asian clades, all of which share common ancestry with the original 1997 Hong Kong strain. Phylogenetic trees built on each of the 8 segments show a consistent picture of 3 lineages. Two of the clades contain exclusively Vietnamese isolates; the smaller of these, with 5 isolates, we label V1; the larger clade, with 9 isolates, is V2.

The remaining 22 isolates all fall into a third, clearly distinct clade, labelled EMA, which comprises samples from Europe, the Middle East, and Africa. Trees for the other 7 segments display a similar topology, with clades V1, V2, and EMA clearly separated in each case. Analyses of all available complete influenza (H5N1) genomes and of 589 HA sequences placed the EMA clade as distinct from the major clades circulating in People's Republic of China, Indonesia, and South East Asia."

Terminology

H5N1 isolates are identified like this actual HPAI A(H5N1) example, A/chicken/Nakorn-Patom/Thailand/CU-K2/04(H5N1):

- A stands for the species of influenza (A, B or C);
- chicken is the species the isolate was found in;
- Nakorn-Patom/Thailand is the place this specific virus was isolated;
- CU-K2 identifies it from other influenza viruses isolated at the same placel
- 04 represents the year 2004;
- H5 stands for the fifth of several known types of the protein hemagglutinin;
- N1 stands for the first of several known types of the protein neuraminidase.

Other examples include: A/duck/Hong Kong/308/78(H5N3), A/avian/NY/01(H5N2), A/chicken/Mexico/31381-3/94(H5N2), and A/shoveler/Egypt/03(H5N2).

As with other avian flu viruses, H5N1 has strains called "highly pathogenic" (HP) and "low-pathogenic" (LP). Avian influenza viruses that cause HPAI are highly virulent, and mortality rates in infected flocks often approach 100 per cent. LPAI viruses have negligible virulence, but these viruses can serve as progenitors to HPAI viruses. The current strain of H5N1 responsible for the deaths of birds across the world is an HPAI strain; all other current strains of H5N1, including a North American strain that causes no disease at all in any species, are LPAI strains. All HPAI strains identified to date have involved H5 and H7 subtypes. The distinction concerns pathogenicity in poultry, not humans. Normally a highly pathogenic avian virus is not highly pathogenic to either humans or non-poultry birds. This current deadly strain of H5N1 is unusual in being deadly to so many species, including some, like domestic cats, never previously susceptible to any influenza virus.

Genetic Structure and Related Subtypes

H5N1 is a subtype of the species *Influenza A virus* of the *Influenzavirus A* genus of the *Orthomyxoviridae* family. Like all other influenza A subtypes, the H5N1 subtype is an RNA virus. It has a segmented genome of eight negative sense, single-strands of RNA, abbreviated as PB2, PB1, PA, HA, NP, NA, MP and NS.

HA codes for hemagglutinin, an antigenic glycoprotein found on the surface of the influenza viruses and is responsible for binding the virus to the cell that is being infected. NA codes for neuraminidase, an antigenic glycosylated enzyme found on the surface of the influenza viruses. It facilitates the release of progeny viruses from infected cells.

The hemagglutinin (HA) and neuraminidase (NA) RNA strands specify the structure of proteins that are most medically relevant as targets for antiviral drugs and antibodies. HA and NA are also used as the basis for the naming of the different subtypes of influenza A viruses. This is where the *H* and *N* come from in *H5N1*.

Influenza A viruses are significant for their potential for disease and death in humans and other animals. Influenza A virus subtypes that have been confirmed in humans, in order of the number of known human pandemic deaths that they have caused, include:

- H1N1, which caused "Spanish flu" and currently causes seasonal human flu
- H2N2, which caused "Asian flu"
- H3N2, which caused "Hong Kong flu" and currently causes seasonal human flu
- H5N1, "Bird Flu," the world's major current pandemic threat
- H7N7, which has unusual zoonotic potential and killed one person
- H1N2, which is currently endemic in humans and pigs and causes seasonal human flu
- H9N2, which has infected three people

- H7N2, which has infected two people
- H7N3, which has infected two people
- H10N7, which has infected two people

Low Pathogenic H5N1

Low pathogenic avian influenza H5N1 (LPAI H5N1) also called "North American" H5N1 commonly occurs in wild birds. In most cases, it causes minor sickness or no noticeable signs of disease in birds. It is not known to affect humans at all. The only concern about it is that it is possible for it to be transmitted to poultry and in poultry mutate into a highly pathogenic strain.

- 1975 – LPAI H5N1 was detected in a wild mallard duck and a wild blue goose in Wisconsin.
- 1981 and 1985 – LPAI H5N1 was detected in ducks by the University of Minnesota conducting a sampling procedure in which sentinel ducks were monitored in cages placed in the wild for a short period of time.
- 1983 – LPAI H5N1 was detected in ring-billed gulls in Pennsylvania.
- 1986 — LPAI H5N1 was detected in a wild mallard duck in Ohio.
- 2005 — LPAI H5N1 was detected in ducks in Manitoba, Canada.
- 2008 — LPAI H5N1 was detected in ducks in New Zealand.
- 2009 — LPAI H5N1 was detected in commercial poultry in British Columbia.

"In the past, there was no requirement for reporting or tracking LPAI H5 or H7 detections in wild birds so states and universities tested wild bird samples independently of USDA. Because of this, the above list of previous detections might not be all inclusive of past LPAI H5N1 detections. However, the World

Organisation for Animal Health (OIE) recently changed its requirement of reporting detections of avian influenza. Effective in 2006, all confirmed LPAI H5 and H7 AI subtypes must be reported to the OIE because of their potential to mutate into highly pathogenic strains. Therefore, USDA now tracks these detections in wild birds, backyard flocks, commercial flocks and live bird markets."

Properties of H5N1

Infectivity: H5N1 is easily transmissible between birds facilitating a potential global spread of H5N1. While H5N1 undergoes mutation and reassortment, creating variations which can infect species not previously known to carry the virus, not all of these variant forms can infect humans. H5N1 as an avian virus preferentially binds to a type of galactose receptors that populate the avian respiratory tract from the nose to the lungs and are virtually absent in humans, occurring only in and around the alveoli, structures deep in the lungs where oxygen is passed to the blood. Therefore, the virus is not easily expelled by coughing and sneezing, the usual route of transmission.

H5N1 is mainly spread by domestic poultry, both through the movements of infected birds and poultry products and through the use of infected poultry manure as fertilizer or feed. Humans with H5N1 have typically caught it from chickens, which were in turn infected by other poultry or waterfowl. Migrating waterfowl (wild ducks, geese and swans) carry H5N1, often without becoming sick. Many species of birds and mammals can be infected with HPAI A(H5N1), but the role of animals other than poultry and waterfowl as disease-spreading hosts is unknown.

According to a report by the World Health Organisation, H5N1 may be spread indirectly. The report stated that the virus may sometimes stick to surfaces or get kicked up in fertilizer dust to infect people.

Virulence: H5N1 has mutated into a variety of strains with differing pathogenic profiles, some pathogenic to one species but not others, some pathogenic to multiple species. Each specific known genetic variation is traceable to a virus isolate of a specific case of infection. Through antigenic drift, H5N1 has mutated into dozens of highly pathogenic varieties divided into genetic clades which are known from specific isolates, but all currently belonging to genotype Z of avian influenza virus H5N1, now the dominant genotype. H5N1 isolates found in Hong Kong in 1997 and 2001 were not consistently transmitted efficiently among birds and did not cause significant disease in these animals. In 2002 new isolates of H5N1 were appearing within the bird population of Hong Kong. These new isolates caused acute disease, including severe neurological dysfunction and death in ducks. This was the first reported case of lethal influenza virus infection in wild aquatic birds since 1961. Genotype Z emerged in 2002 through reassortment from earlier highly pathogenic genotypes of H5N1 that first infected birds in China in 1996, and first infected humans in Hong Kong in 1997. Genotype Z is endemic in birds in South East Asia, has created at least two clades that can infect humans, and is spreading across the globe in bird populations. Mutations are occurring within this genotype that are increasing their pathogenicity. Birds are also able to shed the virus for longer periods of time before their death, increasing the transmissibility of the virus.

Transmission and Host Range

Infected birds transmit H5N1 through their saliva, nasal secretions, feces and blood. Other animals may become infected with the virus through direct contact with these bodily fluids or through contact with surfaces contaminated with them. H5N1 remains infectious after over 30 days at 0°C (32.0°F) (over one month at freezing temperature) or 6 days at 37°C (98.6°F) (one week at human body temperature) so at ordinary temperatures it lasts in the environment for weeks. In Arctic temperatures, it doesn't degrade at all.

Because migratory birds are among the carriers of the highly pathogenic H5N1 virus, it is spreading to all parts of the world. H5N1 is different from all previously known highly pathogenic avian flu viruses in its ability to be spread by animals other than poultry.

In October 2004, researchers discovered that H5N1 is far more dangerous than was previously believed. Waterfowl were revealed to be directly spreading the highly pathogenic strain of H5N1 to chickens, crows, pigeons, and other birds, and the virus was increasing its ability to infect mammals as well. From this point on, avian flu experts increasingly referred to containment as a strategy that can delay, but not ultimately prevent, a future avian flu pandemic.

> "Since 1997, studies of influenza A (H5N1) indicate that these viruses continue to evolve, with changes in antigenicity and internal gene constellations; an expanded host range in avian species and the ability to infect fields; enhanced pathogenicity in experimentally infected mice and ferrets, in which they cause systemic infections; and increased environmental stability."

The New York Times, in an article on transmission of H5N1 through smuggled birds, reports Wade Hagemeijer of Wetlands International stating, "We believe it is spread by both bird migration and trade, but that trade, particularly illegal trade, is more important".

On September 27, 2007 researchers reported that the H5N1 bird flu virus can also pass through a pregnant woman's placenta to infect the fetus. They also found evidence of what doctors had long suspected—that the virus not only affects the lungs, but also passes throughout the body into the gastrointestinal tract, the brain, liver, and blood cells.

High Mutation Rate

Influenza viruses have a relatively high mutation rate that is characteristic of RNA viruses. The segmentation of its genome facilitates genetic recombination by segment reassortment in hosts infected with two different influenza viruses at the same time. A previously uncontagious strain may then be able to pass between humans, one of several possible paths to a pandemic.

The ability of various influenza strains to show species-selectivity is largely due to variation in the hemagglutinin genes. Genetic mutations in the hemagglutinin gene that cause single amino acid substitutions can significantly alter the ability of viral hemagglutinin proteins to bind to receptors on the surface of host cells.

Such mutations in avian H5N1 viruses can change virus strains from being inefficient at infecting human cells to being as efficient in causing human infections as more common human influenza virus types. This doesn't mean that one amino acid substitution can cause a pandemic, but it does mean that one amino acid substitution can cause an avian flu virus that is not pathogenic in humans to become pathogenic in humans.

H3N2 ("Swine influenza") is endemic in pigs in China, and has been detected in pigs in Vietnam, increasing fears of the emergence of new variant strains. The dominant strain of annual flu virus in January 2006 was H3N2, which is now resistant to the standard antiviral drugs amantadine and rimantadine.

The possibility of H5N1 and H3N2 exchanging genes through reassortment is a major concern. If a reassortment in H5N1 occurs, it might remain an H5N1 subtype, or it could shift subtypes, as H2N2 did when it evolved into the Hong Kong Flu strain of H3N2.

Both the H2N2 and H3N2 pandemic strains contained avian influenza virus RNA segments. "While the pandemic human influenza viruses of 1957 (H2N2) and 1968 (H3N2) clearly arose through reassortment between human and avian viruses, the influenza virus causing the 'Spanish flu' in 1918 appears to be entirely derived from an avian source".

Humans and H5N1

The earliest infections of humans by H5N1 coincided with an epizootic (an epidemic in non-humans) of H5N1 influenza in Hong Kong's poultry population. This panzootic (a disease affecting animals of many species, especially over a wide area) outbreak was stopped by the killing of the entire domestic poultry population within the territory.

Symptoms in Humans

The avian influenza hemagglutinin binds alpha 2-3 sialic acid receptors while human influenza haemagglutinins bind alpha 2-6 sialic acid receptors. This means that when the H5N1 strain infects humans it will replicate in the lower respiratory tract, and consequently will cause viral pneumonia. There is as yet no human form of H5N1, so all humans who have caught it so far have caught avian H5N1.

In general, humans who catch a humanised Influenza A virus (a human flu virus of type A) usually have symptoms that include fever, cough, sore throat, muscle aches, conjunctivitis, and, in severe cases, breathing problems and pneumonia that may be fatal. The severity of the infection depends to a large part on the state of the infected person's immune system and whether the victim has been exposed to the strain before (in which case they would be partially immune). No one knows if these or other symptoms will be the symptoms of a humanised H5N1 flu.

The reported mortality rate of highly pathogenic H5N1 avian influenza in a human is high; WHO data indicates that 60 per cent of cases classified as H5N1 resulted in death. However, there is some evidence that the actual mortality rate of avian flu could be much lower, as there may be many people with milder symptoms who do not seek treatment and are not counted.

In one case, a boy with H5N1 experienced diarrhoea followed rapidly by a coma without developing respiratory or flu-like symptoms. There have been studies of the levels of cytokines in humans infected by the H5N1 flu virus. Of particular concern is elevated levels of tumour necrosis factor-alpha, a protein that is associated with tissue destruction at sites of infection and increased production of other cytokines.

Flu virus-induced increases in the level of cytokines is also associated with flu symptoms including fever, chills, vomiting and headache. Tissue damage associated with pathogenic flu virus infection can ultimately result in death.

The inflammatory cascade triggered by H5N1 has been called a 'cytokine storm' by some, because of what seems to be a positive feedback process of damage to the body resulting from immune system stimulation. H5N1 induces higher levels of cytokines than the more common flu virus types.

Treatment and Prevention for Humans

There is no highly effective treatment for H5N1 flu, but oseltamivir (commercially marketed by Roche as Tamiflu), can sometimes inhibit the influenza virus from spreading inside the user's body. This drug has become a focus for some governments and organisations trying to prepare for a possible H5N1 pandemic. On April 20, 2006, Roche AG announced that a stockpile of three million treatment courses of Tamiflu are waiting at the disposal of the World Health Organisation to be used in case of a flu pandemic; separately Roche donated two million courses to the WHO for use in developing nations that may be affected by such a pandemic but lack the ability to purchase large quantities of the drug.

However, WHO expert Hassan al-Bushra has said:

> "Even now, we remain unsure about Tamiflu's real effectiveness. As for a vaccine, work cannot start on it until the emergence of a new virus, and we predict it would take six to nine months to develop it. For the moment, we cannot by any means count on a potential vaccine to prevent the spread of a contagious influenza virus, whose various precedents in the past 90 years have been highly pathogenic".

There are several H5N1 vaccines for several of the avian H5N1 varieties, but the continual mutation of H5N1 renders them of limited use to date: while vaccines can sometimes provide cross-protection against related flu strains, the best protection would be from a vaccine specifically produced for any future pandemic flu virus strain. Dr. Daniel Lucey, co-director of the Biohazardous Threats and Emerging Diseases graduate programme at Georgetown University has made this point, "There is no H5N1 pandemic so there can be no pandemic vaccine". However, "pre-pandemic vaccines" have been created; are being refined and tested; and do have some promise both in furthering research and preparedness for the next pandemic. Vaccine manufacturing companies are being encouraged to increase capacity so that if a pandemic vaccine is needed, facilities will be available for rapid production of large amounts of a vaccine specific to a new pandemic strain.

Animal and lab studies suggest that Relenza (zanamivir), which is in the same class of drugs as Tamiflu, may also be effective against H5N1. In a study performed on mice in 2000, "zanamivir was shown to be efficacious in treating avian influenza viruses H9N2, H6N1, and H5N1 transmissible to mammals". While no one knows if zanamivir will be useful or not on a yet to exist pandemic strain of H5N1, it might be useful to stockpile zanamivir as well as oseltamivir in the event of an H5N1 influenza pandemic. Neither oseltamivir nor zanamivir can currently be manufactured in quantities that would be meaningful once efficient human transmission starts.

In September, 2006, a WHO scientist announced that studies had confirmed cases of H5N1 strains resistant to Tamiflu and Amantadine. Tamiflu-resistant strains have also appeared in the EU, which remain sensitive to Relenza.

11

Swine Flu Outbreak 2009 by Country

This chapter deals with the status and efforts regarding the 2009 swine flu outbreak by country and continent/region.

The Ten Countries with Most Confirmed Cases per Number of Habitants

Pos.	*Country*	*Population*	*Confirmed cases*	*Confirmed cases per 1,000,000 inhabitants*
1	Canada	33,669,000	2,446	72.6
2	Australia	21,714,000	1,207	55.6
3	Panama	3,309,679	179	54.1
4	Chile	16,928,873	890	52.5
5	Mexico	111,157,200	5,717	51.4
6	USA	306,433,000	12,587	41.1
7	Costa Rica	4,000,000	84	21.0
8	UK	58,789,194	621	10.6
9	El Salvador	6,800,000	69	10.1
10	Kuwait	2,700,000	18	6.7
	World	6,783,421,727	25,647	3.8

Affected Countries

Africa:

Benin: Results are expected next week on a European woman who returned from Mexico to Benin showing flu like symptoms.

Egypt: The Egyptian government has increased numbers of medical officers at Cairo Airport and will monitor passengers from Mexico during their stay.

The government ordered the mass slaughter of all pigs in Egypt on April 29, even though the current strain is a human-human transmittable, human influenza that has already previously hybridised with avian and swine flu. The World Organisation for Animal Health called the swine killing "scientifically unjustified".

The first case of the novel H1N1 virus was discovered in Cairo, Egypt on the second of June, in a 12-year-old girl coming from the USA with her mother. Only the girl was infected, and the officials caught the case before getting out of the airport.

Third and Second casses were discovered on Sunday 7th of June, they're 2 students at the American university of Cairo.

As of June 8, there has thus been 3 confirmed case of swine flu in Egypt.

Ghana: Ghana has banned the importation of pork and pork products.

Nigeria: Nigerian Health Minister Babatunde Osotimehin said that the country is stockpiling antiviral treatments, informing the public and increasing surveillance.

South Africa: On April 29, South Africa reported two possible cases of swine flu from two women who had recently travelled in Mexico.

Zambia: An emergency task force has been set up by the Zambian government.

Swine Flu Outbreak in Asia 2009

Azerbaijan: On April 27, Azerbaijan imposed a ban on import of animal husbandry products from America. According to the Chief of the State Veterinary Service under the Agriculture Ministry Ismayil Hasanov, products brought to the country by April 27 received certificates and it was confirmed that those products were safe. AZAL took additional safety measures and a sanitary quarantine unit of the Health Ministry started to operate in Heydar Aliyev International Airport with all aircraft and passengers being checked.

Azeri Minister of Health Ogtay Shiraliyev said the order prepared by him considers implementation of necessary measures in the epidemiological and various medical centres. "Azerbaijan is ready for this issue", he said. According to the Agriculture Minister Ismat Abbasov, the State Veterinary Service is holding monitoring in the regions and pigs are kept in closed places in farms. Abbasov also said: "I can say with full responsibility that the situation on prevention against swine flu virus is stable in Azerbaijan".

On May 2 all checkpoints on borders with Russia passed to the medium security and disinfection barriers for both cars and pedestrians were installed at the Samur, Shirvanovka and Khan Oba checkpoints in Qusar and Khachmaz Raions. The veterinary services at checkpoints intensified their activities while hog farms in the northern regions passed to the closed farming regime.

Cambodia: Cambodia's health authorities remain alert but confident that the country is prepared for a swine flu pandemic. In terms of ensuring that infected pigs do not spread the disease to Cambodia, the Cambodian Pig Raiser Association said it has told the government it should ban live pig imports. But Khlauk Chuon, the deputy director of Camcontrol at the Ministry of Commerce, said they would only ban live pig imports from a country that has been hit with swine flu.

"We are very worried about this new disease because it can transfer from pig to human, from human to human and from human to pig," Khlauk Chuon added.

China: The first suspected case found on mainland China was reported on May 10, 2009.

The General Administration of Quality Supervision, Inspection and Quarantine (AQSIQ) of China issued an emergency notice on the evening of April 26 that visitors returning from flu-affected areas who experienced flu-like symptoms within two weeks would be quarantined. The Ministry of Health has started prevention measures, and initiated cooperation with the WHO and the relevant departments of the Mexican and US governments to help contain the outbreak. According to Wang Jing of the China Inspection and Quarantine Science Research Institute, the measures already in place in China against bird flu are sufficient for this new disease.

May 2, the Chinese government has decided to suspend flights from Mexico to Shanghai, the Foreign Ministry said. Meanwhile, the Civil Aviation Administration of China also assigned a charter to transport stranded Chinese visitors back home. Among all carriers, China Eastern Airlines was the first choice as it is based in Shanghai, where the original and the only Sino-Mexican flight disembarks, but later the job has fallen onto the Guangzhou based China Southern Airlines, as China Eastern's aircrafts don't fit the facility at Tijuana Airport. The replacing China Southern flight would leave Guangzhou at 21:00 on May 3 as a normal flight until it reaches the stop-over at Los Angeles, and then fly empty towards Mexico City to pick up the 120 stranded tourists. The charter flight estimates to be back in Shanghai 11:00 in the morning on May 5, and all passengers onboard will then go through health to see if further action is needed.

Hong Kong: The Food and Health Bureau of Hong Kong issued travel advice for Mexico on April 26, 2009, which advised Hong Kong residents not to travel to Mexico unless absolutely necessary. The first case reported was a Mexican who flew in from Shanghai. The most recent case (the tenth) was found in a 56-year-old American who had flown in from San Francisco.

The Bureau also escalated the alert level from "alert" to "serious" on the same day, which activated health protection measures in all ports of entry of Hong Kong. As such, temperature screening machines are used at all checkpoints to identify passengers with fever and respiratory symptoms.

Any passenger who fails the temperature test and confirmed having a fever will be quarantined and sent to public hospital for further investigation. Hong Kong also became one of the first jurisdictions to declare swine flu as a notifiable disease, and much of the procedures against the spread of the swine flu were learned from the 2003 SARS outbreak, of which Hong Kong was the epicentre of the outbreak.

The Secretary for Food and Health Dr. York Chow stated that special attention will be paid to passengers who come from countries where human infection of swine influenza cases have been reported.

As of April 30, according to the Hong Kong Government, there are no confirmed human case of swine influenza A (H1N1) infections in Hong Kong. There were 9 patients who fulfilled the designated reporting criteria, 8 of which tested negative in swine influenza.

On May 1, one case became the first confirmed case of swine flu in Hong Kong and also the first in Asia after being tested positive by the University of Hong Kong and the Department of Health of Hong Kong. The Mexican patient, who travelled with two companions from Mexico to Hong Kong with a stopover in Shanghai Pudong Airport, arrived in Hong Kong on April 30.

Metropark Hotel Wanchai, where the patient stayed, was cordoned off by the police and health officials from the Centre for Health Protection. All 350 guests and hotel staff have to remain inside the hotel for seven days. After the first swine flu case was confirmed by laboratory, Chief Executive Sir Donald Tsang raised Hong Kong's response level from "serious" to "emergency".

On May 2, a total of 12 Metropark Hotel guests who were not willing to stay in the hotel were moved to Lady MacLehose Holiday Village in Sai Kung for quarantine.

India: The Government of India has decided to screen all people entering India via the main airport hubs of Mumbai, New Delhi, Goa, Jaipur, Kochi, Chennai, Bangalore and Hyderabad. It said the primary focus will be on passengers entering from the United States of America, The United Kingdom, Canada, Mexico, France, and New Zealand. A team of 32 medical professionals have been posted at these airports. The Ministry of Health is also trying to track down people who have entered India from Mexico in the last 10 days. It has been reported that one person recently travelled from Texas to Hyderabad with flu symptoms and was quarantined, but authorities refused to divulge his identity. Government health officials and WHO subsequently stated that there is no Swine flu in India and the said patient recovered from a common cold. Three other suspected cases of swine flu have been noticed. Two of them were flying from Chicago and the other one, who is UK citizen, aged 35, arrived from London. All of whom have been kept under observation in a hospital. As of June 6 2009, Five cases have been confirmed in India

Indonesia: After a coordination meeting about the flu on April 27, 2009, the Indonesian government halted the importation of pigs and initiated the examination of 9 million pigs in Indonesia. Thermal scanners which can detect human body temperature have been installed at Indonesian ports of entry. Temperatures above 38°C (100.4°F) cause the devices to beep, indicating fever. The devices have been installed in Soekarno-Hatta International Airport and Halim Perdana Kusuma Airport in Jakarta, Juanda Airport in Surabaya, Hang Nadim Airport in Batam, Hasanudin Airport in Makassar, Ngurah Rai Airport in Denpasar, Sepinggan Airport in Balikpapan, and Tanjung Priok Seaport, gates one and two in Jakarta and taking action right now.

Israel: Thirty-three cases have been confirmed in Israel. In response to the outbreak, the Israeli Deputy Minister of Health, Yaakov Litzman, has said that because *swine* are unclean, the outbreak needs to be renamed, and so in Israel, out of respect for the religious sensibilities of Jews and Muslims, it should be called "Mexican Flu". This was done so as to not confuse the population into thinking that they could not acquire the virus if they did not eat pork. The Israeli government retracted this proposal following Mexican complaints.

Japan: The Ministry of Agriculture, Forestry and Fisheries of Japan instructed animal quarantine offices across Japan to examine any live pigs being brought into Japan to make sure they are not infected with the influenza. Japanese Agriculture Minister Shigeru Ishiba appeared on television to reassure customers that it is safe to eat pork. The Japanese farm ministry said that it would not ask for restrictions on pork imports because the virus was unlikely to turn up in pork, and would be killed by cooking.

On 30 April 2009, the first suspected case was detected at Narita Airport. However, the case turned out to be a conventional strain of influenza A subtype H3N2 (Hong Kong A strain). On 1 May 2009, the second suspected case was detected in Yokohama. This case also turned out to be a conventional strain of influenza A subtype H1N1 (Russian A strain). Meanwhile Japan has not stopped any flights or means of travelling between Japan and Mexico.

On 8 May, the first three cases were confirmed. The infected patients had spent time in Oakville, Canada and returned to Japan via Detroit. On 10 May, another case was confirmed from a student who came from a school trip to Canada, making it the fourth case of Japan.

On 16 May, the first domestic infection was confirmed in Kobe. The male high school student did not have a history of travel abroad and thought it was a seasonal flu, and PCR test was not done in timely manner. Two other students are suspected, and 17 other students are claiming influenza-like symptoms. The route of the infection was not traceable.

On 18 May, 130 cases had been confirmed, including employees of a railway kiosk and a bank. Several railway kiosks in Kobe were closed, and 70 other bank workers who had worked with the infected person were told to stand by at home. All schools in the Osaka and Hyogo Prefectures were suspended.

Kuwait: About 18 people on US military bases in Kuwait have tested positive for swine flu, a US Central Command spokeswoman said Friday.

They are the first cases reported in Kuwait. It remains unclear whether the virus has spread to the civilian population.

The names and units of the infected people were not immediately available.

Maj. Kristi Beckman, speaking from Central Command headquarters in Tampa, said everyone who tested positive for the virus was quarantined in military health facilities approved by officials from the Kuwaiti Ministry of Health.

The World Health Organisation reported about H1N1 influenza did not include Kuwait on its list of countries where the virus is present. Kuwait is used as a staging area for soldiers heading to or from the war in Iraq.

On April 28, the Kuwait Times newspaper reported that the country was free of the virus.

The country is aggressively screening anyone arriving in Kuwait to prevent the virus from entering the country, Beckman said. Anyone who exhibits symptoms of the illness is immediately isolated and tested using WHO and Centres for Disease Control guidelines, Beckman said.

"The embassy in Kuwait has been working with the Kuwait Ministry of Health and other US military elements in Kuwait just to assure we're safeguarding the health of all residents in Kuwait," Beckman said.

The US has about 135,000 troops fighting in Iraq, Kuwait's northern neighbour. About 4,000 soldiers from the 30th Heavy Brigade Combat Team of the North Carolina National Guard deployed to Iraq last month. And about 3,500 paratroopers from the 82nd Airborne Division's 3rd Brigade Combat Team started a yearlong deployment to Iraq in December.

Laos: The Lao government agreed to buy 10 thermal imaging machines and install them at the country's major immigration border checkpoints. The machines would help officials identify anyone entering the country with a high temperature and create confidence among Lao people, foreigners living in Laos and people travelling to Laos. Health officials would be on hand at international border checkpoints to ensure anyone found to be infected could be treated immediately. Each machine could cost about US $25,000. The decision to buy them was made after the government found visitors to Laos included people coming from the United States, Spain and other affected countries.

The machines would help officials identify anyone entering the country with a high temperature and create confidence among Lao people, foreigners living in Laos and people travelling to Laos. Health officials would be on hand at international border checkpoints to ensure anyone found to be infected could be treated immediately.

Lebanon: Three cases of swine flu have been diagnosed in Lebanon (30 May 2009), the first in the country, Health Minister Mohammad Jawad Khalifeh announced on Saturday. "One Lebanese man who was in Spain and two Canadians who arrived in Lebanon a week ago are suffering from swine flu," Khalifeh told AFP. "We put them in quarantine and the blood samples we have taken every day have proven to be positive. "The Lebanese man and the two visiting Canadians — a woman and her daughter — were given the proper medical treatment in time and they are well now." He told a press conference said the man was part of a group of 22 Lebanese who had been attending a training seminar in Spain at an institute where the disease was later detected. "That prompted us to check all the passengers on board the plane on which the group was returning and one case was detected," Khalifeh said. He added that the virus was not homegrown and came from abroad. "We are going to have to take additional measures," he said. "We are going to take more precautions at the airport." He said health authorities may use thermal scanners at the airport to detect passengers with fever. "The situation is under control," he said.

The Lebanese Health Minister Mohammad Jawad Khalifeh asked citizens to stop the social habit of greeting with kissing, as it is a Lebanese habit to greet each other with three kisses on the cheek. He also requested that affected schoolchildren be kept at home and that travel to countries in which cases have been confirmed be avoided. Beirut also banned the import of pork.

On May 30, Lebanon confirms three cases of swine flu.

Malaysia: According to the Malaysian Ministry of Health, headed by Liow Tiong Lai, health screenings were carried out on passengers travelling to and from Mexico via sea, air and land beginning April 17. The Health Ministry's disease control division has activated its operations room to monitor the swine flu situation and informed medical practitioners who are treating cases with symptoms of influenza-like illness or severe pneumonia and persons who had visited Mexico, California or Texas to inform the district health office immediately for preventive and control measures. As has several Asian countries, thermal scanners had been installed at entry points at the Kuala Lumpur International Airport (KLIA) following the start of the global alert on the flu. Screenings were imposed in Pengkalan Hulu, at the border with Thailand, in late-April. Quarantine rooms had been allocated in 28 hospitals, and the country has stockpiled more than 2 million doses of Tamilflu, as of May 2009.

In response to the country's first case of A (H1N1), the health ministry urged calm among the populace "as the situation is under control" and "the ministry has taken all the possible precautionary measures to control and contain the disease after the WHO issued a level-five alert." In addition, schools were issued strict hygiene procedures on May 16 to contain any H1N1 outbreak among students and teachers.

The country had reported no suspected cases before May 4, 2009, but all cases tested negative between May 4 and May 15. On May 15, the Health Ministry confirmed Malaysia's first case of A (H1N1) infection of a 21 year-old male student who had arrived at the KLIA on May 13 via a Malaysia Airlines flight (MH091) from Newark and on transit at Stockholm-Arlanda Airport, followed by a second case on May 16 of a female student in Penang who shared the same flight as the first victim and boarded an AirAsia flight (AK5358) from KLIA to Penang International Airport. This makes Malaysia the 36th country to detect A (H1N1) within its borders.

The first victim has been warded at the Sungai Buloh Hospital, while house quarantines were undertaken on two of the second victim's friends who boarded the same flight, along with their family members. All passengers of the flights were also asked to contact the Health Ministry or head to any hospital, clinic or health office or further action, and crew members of MH091 and AK5358 were located and grounded. As the first victim has indicated, the use of thermal scanners is revealed not to be entirely effective as symptoms of his flu had yet to manifest; the Health Ministry resumes the use of the scanners nevertheless.

On June 4, three additional inbound airline passengers were reported to be carrying the virus. The earliest of the three is a 23-year-old male student who returned from United States on June 1 via the same Malaysian Airlines flight (MH091) that the first cases of A (H1N1) were detected. On the same day, two German tourists and friends (aged 30 and 32) who were holidaying in South East Asia and arrived in Malaysia were confirmed to be infected with the virus; both had flown into the country on June 3 via an Air Asia flight (AK702) after transferring from a Singapore Airlines flight (SQ45) from Germany to Singapore on June 1. The third reported victim developed symptoms on June 3 and was warded in Tunku Jaafar Hospital, while the two tourists developed symptoms while in Kuala Lumpur on June 3 and were given similar medical treatment. All three victims were reported to be stable. As is has been for the last two cases, passengers sharing both the Malaysian Airlines and Air Asia flights are being traced. On June 5, sixth case were reported from a student who took the same flight with the fourth patient. On the next day, a girl from Australia was confirmed to be infected with Influenza A (H1N1) when the airport scanner detected severe fever making her the 7th confirmed case overall in Malaysia.

Maldives: A ministerial committee has been established to supervise swine flu preventive measures to avoid an outbreak. All visitors arriving at the Malé International Airport on Hulhule Island and the country's three commercial seaports are being screened.

Myanmar: Deputy Health Minister inspects human flu preventive measures at airport YANGON, May 1-Chairman of Global Human Flu Prevention and Response Work Committee Deputy Minister for Health Dr. Mya Oo inspected preventive measures against the human flu at Yangon International Airport today.

Pakistan: Pakistan has taken precautionary measures at the international airports to check passengers coming from swine flu affected countries. Doctors are checking the incoming passengers and allow entry only to those with no flu symptoms. The major hospitals in all the big cities are on high alert.

Philippines: Health Secretary Francisco T. Duque III ordered the Bureau of Quarantine to use thermal imaging equipment at airports to screen passengers coming from the US for flu symptoms. The Philippines may quarantine travellers arriving from Mexico with fevers. Also, the Secretary of the Department of Agriculture issued an order banning the importation of hogs from the US and Mexico, and the retraction of the restriction of swine influenza vaccine use. The medical alert phase is already Code White, the lowest.

On May 18, 2009, a Filipina girl who arrived from the US was the first confirmed case of H1N1 virus in the Philippines. Health Secretary Duque advised that the girl is in stable condition and is in quarantine.

On June 3, 2009, a foreign exchange student in De La Salle University-Manila was confirmed with H1N1 virus and the school was closed for ten days starting June 4.

As of June 5, 2009, the Total of confirmed cases of A(H1N1) virus rose from 29 cases last June 4 to 33 confirmed cases as of June 5. Philippine Health Secretary Francisco Duque III said the new cases are two siblings and another student of De La Salle University.

Because of the said incident, on June 6, 2009, the Commission in Higher Education (CHED) moved the opening of classes in all colleges and universities in Metro Manila from June 8, 2009 to June 15, 2009.

Saudi Arabia: The Health Ministry has announced detection of a case of swine flu which affected a Filipino nurse working at King Faisal Specialist Hospital and Research Centre. Dr. Abdullah al-Rabee'a, the Health Minister said the detection of the case has come within the framework of the efforts being exerted by the Health Ministry to follow up developments in this respect. In a statement to the Saudi Press Agency, he said the nurse, who had spent her holidays in Philippines, returned to Riyadh on Friday, May 29, 2009, aboard one of the flights of the Gulf Air." Symptoms of the disease appeared in the case of the nurse on Monday June 1, 2009, and she was admitted to the KFSHRC for conducting the required medical examinations pertaining to Swine Flu, he said, noting that the results of the medical examinations were disclosed on Tuesday evening, confirming the case as "Positive". In the light of the measures of the World Health Organisation (WHO) the medical examinations were conducted for the second time on Tuesday evening, he said, adding that the examinations proved the infection of the nurse for A/H-I N-I on Wednesday morning. Dr. Al-Rabee'a said the Health Ministry in cooperation with King Faisal Specialist Hospital and Research Centre has applied the national plan for the prevention of Swine Flu in a manner that matches with the recommendations of WHO. Accordingly, the patient was isolated and provided with the required medical treatment. Arrangements are underway to examine those who were in contact with the patient to get sure that they are not infected.

Singapore: The first case of Influenza A (H1N1-2009) was confirmed on May 27, 2009 in Singapore. As of June 6 there were 15 confirmed cases.

South Korea: South Korea warned against travel to Mexico City and three Mexican states. The government has also stepped up quarantine and safety checks on travellers arriving from the United States and Mexico, and pork imports from those countries. An emergency quarantine system is also in place, with simple tests conducted on people arriving with flu symptoms at airports. On April 28, South Korea reported its first probable case of swine flu after positive preliminary tests on a nun who had recently returned from a trip to Mexico. Several sources have informed that one case has been confirmed by lab in South Korea, on April 30. On May 2, the first suspected woman turned out to be infected with the influenza A subtype H1N1. South Korea became the second infected nation in Asia.

Taiwan: On May 20, 2009, the first case of the influenza has been confirmed in Taiwan.

The government had previously taken several steps to prevent the possible outbreak of Swine Flu, including a command centre set up, travel alerts for infected nations, and more severe health check been conducted at international ports. Taiwan said visitors who came back from affected areas with fevers would be quarantined. According to The Department of Health (DOH), Taiwan has a sufficient supply of surgical masks and vaccine to deal with the flu. The DOH also stated that they have 50 million to 60 million masks in stock and local manufacturers have the capability of producing 200,000 doses of the flu vaccine a month. In an effort to prevent the entry of the swine influenza, the Centres for Disease Control has announced on April 28 that every flight from the Americas, specifically Canada and the United States, that arrives in Taiwan from April 29 and onward will be subject to a strict on-board screening procedure.

Thailand: On Tuesday, May 13th, 2009 Thailand confirmed two cases of swine flu. Both of the individuals confirmed as having swine flu had recently travelled to Mexico. By June 2nd there had been five cases of swine flu identified in Thailand.

Vietnam: Vietnam's Ministry of Health released an emergency dispatch and urged agencies to take precautionary measures against swine flu. In addition, the Preventive Health and Environment Bureau requested all health facilities to carefully monitor any suspected H1N1 case and Bureau head Nguyen Huy Nga also warned that the pandemic could enter Vietnam through imported swine or border gates. Thermal imaging devices were dispatched to airports and border gates to screen passengers. In response to WHO's warnings, Vietnam on April 30, 2009 raised its swine flu alert level to 4 which indicated a "threat of community level outbreaks" while local authorities have been executing precautionary measures.

On May 1, 2009 an Vietnam's Ministry of Industry and Trade official said that Ministry was considering a ban on pork import "under certain situations" to prevent swine flu from entering Vietnam.

As of May 31, 2009. The Government of Vietnam announced its First new case of A(H1N1) virus in the Country. A 23 years old Vietnamese student who recently returned from the United States has tested positive for swine flu.

Western and Central Asia

On April 27, Azerbaijan imposed a ban on import of animal husbandry products from America. AZAL took additional safety measures and a sanitary quarantine unit of the Health

Ministry started to operate in Heydar Aliyev International Airport with all aircraft and passengers being checked.

Thirty-three cases have been confirmed in Israel. In response to the outbreak, the Israeli Deputy Minister of Health, Yaakov Litzman, has said that because *swine* are unclean, the outbreak needs to be renamed, and so in Israel, out of respect for the religious sensibilities of Jews and Muslims, it should be called "Mexican Flu". This was done so as to not confuse the population into thinking that they could not acquire the virus if they did not eat pork. The Israeli government retracted this proposal following Mexican complaints.

The first confirmed cases of swine flu in Kuwait were reported on May 23, after about 18 people on US military bases tested positive.

On May 30, three cases of swine flu were confirmed in Lebanon, the first in the country. "One Lebanese man who was in Spain and two Canadians who arrived in Lebanon a week ago are suffering from swine flu," the health minister said. "We put them in quarantine and the blood samples we have taken every day have proven to be positive. The Lebanese man and the two visiting Canadians — a woman and her daughter — were given the proper medical treatment in time and they are well now." The Lebanese Health Minister had previously asked citizens to stop the social habit of kissing. He also requested that affected schoolchildren be kept at home and that travel to countries in which cases have been confirmed be avoided. Beirut also banned the import of pork.

In Saudi Arabia, the first case of swine flu, which affected a Filipino nurse working at King Faisal Specialist Hospital and Research Centre, was confirmed on June 1. The Health Ministry in cooperation with King Faisal Specialist Hospital and Research Centre has applied the national plan for the prevention of Swine Flu in a manner that matches with the recommendations of WHO. Accordingly, the patient was isolated and provided with the required medical treatment. Arrangements are underway to examine those who were in contact with the patient to get sure that they are not infected.

Swine Flu Outbreak in Europe 2009

European Union: On April 27, the European Union health commissioner advised Europeans not to travel to the United States or Mexico unless urgent. This followed the discovery of the first confirmed case in Spain.

EU Foreign relations commissioner Benita Ferrero-Waldner said on April 29 the halt of all travel to Mexico and disinfecting all airports due to the global flu outbreak is being considered.

Austria: Several possible cases in Austria turned out to be negative, whereas one test, that of a 28-year-old woman from Vienna, had a positive result. Therefore, Austria is the 9th country affected by a confirmed case of swine flu. There are still two suspected cases being tested.

Belgium: Six suspected cases of swine flu in Belgium ultimately tested negative.

The Belgian interior ministry announced the first case of A/H1N1 flu in Belgium on 13 May 2009. The infected person is a 28-year-old man who lives in Ghent and returned from a holiday in the United States.

Also a second person tested positive for Mexican flu in Belgium on 14 May 2009.

Two new persons tested positive for A/H1N1 flu on 15 May 2009.

A sixth and seventh case of swine flu was discovered on 21 May 2009. An eighth infection was reported on 26 May 2009.

Bulgaria: The first case of swine flu was a person from New York to Sofia on the 27th May. The person developed respiratory problems, cough and high fever on the 29th May.

Croatia: On April 29 it was announced that a 22-year-old traveller from Florida had been held in quarantine in Osijek under suspicion of swine flu. However, later that day director of infectious disease epidemiology agency, Dr. Ira Gjenero Margan, stated results of the testing were negative "with

99 per cent certainty". On April 30, a child was held in quarantine in Zagreb but the results were negative.

Cyprus: Cyprus has identified its first case of the new H1N1 flu virus on May 30. The patient was a 39-year-old woman from Moldova, living in Cyprus, who returned from the United States on May 28.

Denmark: Authorities confirmed on May 1 that a Danish citizen had tested positive for swine flu, making it the first reported case in Scandinavia.

Estonia: The first case was Laboratory confirmed on May 29. The patient was a 29-year-old man, who returned from the United States. On June 3, two new cases have been Laboratory confirmed.

Finland: The H1N1 strain of influenza has been added to the official list of infectious diseases dangerous to public (yleisvaarallinen tartuntatauti), which guarantees free-of-charge treatment to all residents and allows for involuntary quarantine, effective from May 1 2009. Finland's first two H1N1-cases confirmed 12.5.2009 in Helsinki metropolitan area. They were together in Mexico and came to Finland via Amsterdam 6.5.2009.

France: As of April 28 there were twenty suspected cases of swine flu being investigated in France. Since April 25, over 100 cases of Influenza-like illness have been reported, of which 30 were identified as possible cases. 10 of those cases have since been excluded. On April 30, the number of suspected cases was revised to 50 (including 4 probable cases).

On May 1, the French Health Minister has confirmed, during the 8 pm TF1 news, that 2 cases of A(H1N1) flu have been detected in France.

On May 4, two new cases have been confirmed bringing to 4 the total number of people infected.

May 6, a fifth case is confirmed in Paris region. Two new cases are also confirmed at the end of the afternoon by the

INVS (National Institute for Sanitary Watch), 7 are probable and 32 are suspected.

On May 7, three new cases were announced by the National Institute for Sanitary Watch. There are now 10 confirmed cases, 5 probable, and 27 are suspected.

Germany: On April 29, the first case of swine flu in Germany was confirmed by the Robert Koch Institute in the area of Regensburg.

On May 1, Robert Koch Institute confirmed the first case of human-to-human spreading of swine flu in Munich. Infected was the nurse who had contact with one of the infected people.

Until 5 June, 2009, the total number of confirmed cases increased to 49. Most of them have been recent travellers to Mexico, the US or the UK. However, there was also a single-digit number of (isolated) in-country-transmissions.

Greece: On 19 May 2009 the authorities confirmed the first case of the new flu in Greece. The infected person is a 19-year-old Greek student who studies in New York and who flew to Greece a few days ago. He is hospitalised at Sismanogleion but is not gravely ill. The authorities have contacted many of the passengers who sat near this patient on the plane and are examining them for suspicious symptoms. At this point in time Greece has enough antivirals to cover 12 per cent of the population (at least 10 per cent is the amount proposed by the EU directives). The 19-year-old is now out of the hospital and none of the passengers in his flight are infected.

On 29 May 2009 the fourth case was announced.

Hungary: According to the MTI as of April 29 six suspected cases have been reported in Hungary, none of them confirmed to be the swine flu. Samples of the virus from the US health authorities are due to arrive to Hungary in a few days enabling the start of vaccine production.

On May 29, a case has been confirmed. The infected person, a Brazilian man has since recovered and left the country.

Iceland: The first case of A(H1N1) in Iceland was reported on May 23, 2009. The infected person came to the country from New York and got sick shortly after he arrived in Iceland. It is suspected that additional four people might be infected. All the cases are within the same family and they are located in the Greater Reykjavik area and Sudurland regions.

Iceland is currently being briefed by the WHO and is cooperating closely with ECDC, CDC and the EU in terms of monitoring and response. Initially the directorate of health warned people travelling to Mexico and the United States (especially California and Texas) to exercise caution and to contact a doctor immediately if they started showing symptoms of swine flu but on April 28 people travelling to Mexico were advised to cancel their trip unless its very urgent.

On April 28, it was announced that passengers arriving in Iceland from the United States or Mexico would be monitored and will undergo medical examination even if the slightest signs of influenza are detected.

Iceland has stocks of Tamiflu and Relenza for one-third of its population.

In a risk assessment made by the Icelandic government in 2008 in case of a influenza pandemic two scenarios are envisioned:

- A worst-case scenario where 50 per cent of the Icelandic population are infected and 3 per cent of the infected population die.
- A milder scenario where precautionary measures prevent infection, 25 per cent of the Icelandic population are infected and 1 per cent die.

Ireland: Ireland has over two million doses of antivirals and a pandemic plan in place.

On May 2, the Department of Health's (HSE) announced the first confirmed case in Ireland, an adult male living in Dublin who had recently been to Mexico.

From 25 May to 31 May, three more cases were confirmed.

On 2 June, 3 new cases were confirmed by the HSE on people who returned recently from New York. This brings the total of people in Ireland with Swine Flu to 7.

Italy: Italy's agriculture lobby, Coldiretti, warned against panic reaction, noting that farmers lost hundreds of millions of euros due to consumer boycotts during the 2001 mad cow scare and the 2005 bird flu outbreak.

A woman who returned from San Diego was hospitalised in Venice for suspected swine flu.

As of April 30, about 20 suspected cases of swine flu are monitored in Italy.

On May 2, Reuters confirmed that Italy had a case of the swine flu. It was recorded in a 50-year-old man in Massa after he returned from Mexico City. However, he had very mild symptoms (i.e. aches, coughing, but no fever) and is recovering well.

Lithuania: As of April 29, one possible case (tourist returned from Mexico) in Lithuania is currently under investigation. The institutions already confirmed that it is the A type influenza, but the details as to whether it is H1N1 are still not known. For further investigation sample was sent to the laboratory located in London.

Macedonia: On April 27 2009, the government of the Republic of Macedonia prohibited all exports and imports of live pigs. Even though Macedonia is not affected from the Swine Flu, the government ordered a ten days health monitoring period for everybody that comes from an affected country.

Netherlands: The Netherlands National Institute for Public Health and the Environment advised any traveller who returned from Mexico since April 17 and developed a fever of 38.5°C (101.3°F) within four days of arriving in the Netherlands to stay at home. On April 30, 2009 a three-year-old child tested positive for the swine flu. The child returned from Mexico to the Netherlands on April 27, 2009. The parents tested negative to the swine flu. The girl was very ill at first according to her parents, but made a full recovery. On 7 May a second case and a day later a third case of swine flu in the Netherlands were announced, concerning a 53-year-old woman and a 52-year-old man, respectively. Both of them had returned from Mexico recently and are being treated with Tamiflu. The woman made a full recovery, the man is doing well. There are no connections between each of the three cases. People who were seated close to the infected people in the plane were contacted and are being treated with Tamiflu as a precautionary measure.

Norway: On May 9, two Norwegian students from Oslo and Telemark, were confirmed to be infected with swine flu after they came home from studies in Mexico. None of them became seriously ill and they are recovering quickly. A member of one of their families is suspected of being infected as well. One of them (the 20 year-old man from Oslo) have been confirmed completely recovered. These are the first two cases of swine influenza in Norway.

On June 4, a Norwegian woman from Vest-Agder who recently had been to the United States was confirmed with the swine influenza. The infected woman is recovering well. This is the ninth confirmed case of swine influenza.

Poland: As of May 28, Poland has four confirmed cases — one of which a 58-year-old woman from Mielec, who came back from the USA. She was already released from the hospital, because all of her symptoms had been successfully cured . As of May 8, eight cases are under investigation, according to the National Institute of Public Health and news channel TVN 24. At least 19 other patients had been previously investigated but tests turned out negative. The Polish Foreign Ministry issued a statement on April 25 or earlier recommending that citizens avoid travel to affected areas until the outbreak is totally contained.

Portugal: As of May 4, there has been one confirmed case in Lisbon, Portugal, but it did not represent any preoccupation, because the risk of transmission was no longer present at that time.

On June 1, Ana Jorge, the Portuguese minister of health, has confirmed the second case in Portugal. A 33-year-old man who travelled from the United States, first landing in Frankfurt, Germany, the case was reported at Sao Joao Hospital, Oporto.

Romania: In Sambateni, Arad County, a child of a year and six months and his mother who recently returned from a trip to Portugal and Spain were suspected of having contracted influenza A(H1N1). Tests returned negative. On Wednesday, 27 May a woman returning from America was confirmed with swine flu in Bucharest.

Russia: Russia has banned the import of pork meat from Guatemala, Honduras, Dominican Republic, Colombia, Costa Rica, Cuba, Nicaragua, Panama, El Salvador, 9 US States (Alabama, Arizona, Arkansas, Georgia, Kansas, Louisiana, New Mexico, Oklahoma and Florida) and all types of meat and meat products from Mexico and 5 US States (California, Texas, Kansas, New York and Ohio).

The President instructed the regional governors to take urgent steps to prevent swine flu from spreading to Russia. Dmitry Medvedev also instructed the presidential plenipotentiary envoys in the federal districts to personally supervise the preventive measures to ensure the disease did not spread [in Russia] and stipulated monthly reports on the situation.

On May 1 officials confirmed that two women who came from USA trip were suspected to have swine flu. Currently both are in hospital for further treatment. As on May 2, both tourists are reported not to be infected with new strain.

Serbia: According to Deputy Health Minister Svetlana Mijatovic, Serbia will adhere to all WHO recommendations for monitoring the swine flu epidemic. "A sanitary inspection, together with Serbian Ministry of Internal Affairs (MUP), is checking travellers, [...] while the media and all the agencies throughout the world, as well as our own, are constantly informing the public that if anyone feels ill, or is coming from a contaminated area, to consult the authorities at any airport in the world [...]," Mijatovic said. Serbia's Health Minister stated on May 8, 2009 that there have been no registered cases of swine flu, and that Serbia has stockpiles of antiviral medicine, although he admitted it would not stop a pandemic of swine flu in that country.

Flights and holidays to Mexico and the US have yet to be cancelled, and the advice to citizens travelling to infected countries is to take precautions in terms of immunity and to maintain personal hygiene.

A 71-year-old tourist from Texas asked to be tested for swine flu at the Provincial hospital in Novi Sad, on April 30. Results were negative.

Slovenia: *Institute of Public Health of the Republic of Slovenia* has established a website with information about H1N1 induced influenza. Status of this webpage is updated once a day. As of May 25, there were 17 people tested, all negative.

Spain: On April 27 the Spanish Ministry of Health and Social Policy announced that a man in Castilla-La Mancha who had recently returned from Mexico had contracted the disease. The man, aged 23, had returned from Mexico on April 22 and had been quarantined on the 25th. This was the first confirmed case in Europe.

The Spanish government is also observing other 35 possible swine flu cases in the Basque Country, Catalonia, the Balearic Islands, Andalusia, Murcia, Madrid and the Valencian Community.

AENA, the Spanish state owned company who manages all Spanish airports and Air Traffic Control established a protocol for the flights coming from and to Spain from the affected areas. Three patients who had just returned from Mexico were under observation in multiple regions of Spain.

Sweden: On April 28, at least eighteen Swedish people were tested for swine flu after returning from trips in Mexico and the USA, but the results were negative. On April 29 two people, recently returned from Mexico with flu like symptoms were tested.

As of May 6, the Swedish Institute for Infectious Disease Control confirms 1 case of influenza A(H1N1). 186 negative test results have been reported. No suspected cases remain to be analysed.

The number of confirmed cases has reached 2 in Sweden, with 435 negative cases reported as of May 15.

A third case was confirmed on Friday 15, and reported on the following Saturday, where the patient, a woman in her sixties, has recovered. In all of the 3 cases the influenza was contracted in the USA.

A fourth case was confirmed 28 May, influenza contracted in USA.

Switzerland: The first suspicious case was officially confirmed on April 27. A young man returning from holiday in Mexico informed his family doctor about fever and flu-like symptoms. He was immediately put under quarantine in a hospital. 8 more people are under observation. A container of inactive swine flu virus samples packed in dry ice exploded on a Swiss train, injuring one person but posing no other risks to humans.

Switzerland has confirmed its first case of swine flu in a 19-year-old student who returned from Mexico on April 30. The state hospital in Baden said in a statement that the National Influenza Centre in Geneva confirmed the disease shortly after the student was mistakenly released from hospital day before.

Switzerland has confirmed its second case of swine flu in a young woman of 24. She was returning from a trip to Mexico and USA. She is now in the Hospital in Bern.

On May 24, a third case of swine flu has been announced in a woman who came back from Washington. She is in Basel at home.

As of June 5, there are 14 confirmed cases in seven cantons.

Turkey: The Government of Turkey has taken measures at the international airports, using thermal imaging cameras to check passengers coming from international destinations. . Turkey confirmed its first case of swine flu on May 16 in a US tourist arriving into the country.

Ukraine: Imports of pork and live pigs from all affected countries have been banned. The ban also applies to all shipments after April 21. On June 5, 2009 the first case of the virus was officially confirmed in Ukraine. The patient concerned, a 24-year-old Ukrainian citizen, had arrived from New York via Paris at Kyiv's Boryspil Airport on May 29, 2009.

United Kingdom: Samples from suspected cases have been analysed by the National Institute for Medical Research in London, which is also examining samples of the US strain of the disease.

The first cases were confirmed on 27 April in passengers returning from Mexico. The first case of person to person transmission within the UK was announced on 1 May.

On May 1 the first UK person to person transmission was confirmed. Graeme Pacitti, 24, of Falkirk, picked up the virus after contact with the UK's first cases Iain and Dawn Askham.

It was reported on 26 May that a man who has been confirmed of swine flu is critically ill, since then 4 more people have become critically ill due to swine flu in the UK all in Scotland.

On 28 May, people at a Home Office building in Sheffield were quarantined, it was feared someone had caught Swine Flu on a recent trip to Canada. In fact, not one, but three people had caught it, the person who had been to Canada, one from someone who recently had stayed in Acapulco, Mexico, and one from someone who recently had stayed in London.

On 6 June, the total of swine flu cases hit 508 with 3 people in intensive care in hospital. On 7 June, the total of swine flu cases hit 541 with 3 people in intensive care and one woman with Swine Flu gave birth in hospital.

Swine Flu Outbreak in the United States 2009

The United States (US) experienced an outbreak of Influenza A virus subtype H1N1, commonly known as the swine flu, in the spring of 2009. The outbreak apparently spread from an earlier outbreak in Mexico. Initial US infections occurred in late-March 2009 in California, and by mid-April had spread to scores of people across several states. Public health officials in the United States and the World Health Organisation (WHO) expressed serious concern because the initial outbreak was suspected in over 100 deaths in Mexico, transmitted easily from person to person, and no vaccine was available, prompting President Obama to declare a public health emergency.

By the end of April, hundreds of people were confirmed or suspected as infected, one person had died, and hundreds of schools were closed, keeping over 161,000 students at home. Experts were puzzled by the fact that nearly all the deaths were in Mexico, even though the flu had spread to thousands of others across the world, and that it disproportionately infected young people. By early-May, however, public health officials expressed cautious optimism that the infection was relatively mild and was not spreading as quickly as initially feared. The Centres for Disease Control and Prevention (CDC) issued new guidance, and most schools across the country quickly reopened. Even so, officials cautioned that the flu might mutate and return with more severe consequences during the fall flu season. The CDC is continuously monitoring the ongoing outbreak, and the US Food and Drug Administration (FDA) is currently working on a vaccine for the fall flu season.

As of May 25, the CDC reports that there have been a total of 6,764 human cases of H1N1 infection in the United States. Tallies of cases reported by other public health agencies result in higher figures, and the head of flu epidemiology for the CDC has postulated that the actual number of cases is "upwards of 100,000" as patients with mild cases are not likely to be tested.

As of May 21 the outbreak had spread to 47 states and the District of Columbia, however with over 5000 confirmed or probable cases, only 10 deaths have been confirmed. In a press briefing on May 20, Dr. Daniel Jernigan of the CDC stated, that 247 individuals had been hospitalised and over 70 per cent of those patients had underlying chronic medical conditions, including pregnancy, asthma and heart disease.

Initial Cases

The Centres for Disease Control and Prevention (CDC) identified the first two A/09(H1N1) swine flu cases in California on April 17, 2009 via the Border Infectious Disease Programme, for the San Diego County child, and a naval research facility studying a special diagnostic test, where influenza sample from the child from Imperial County was tested. By April 21, enhanced surveillance was established to search for additional cases in both California and Texas and the CDC determined that the virus strain was genetically similar to the previously known A(H1N1) swine flu circulating among pigs in the United States since about 1999.

It was established that the virus was a combination of human, North American swine, and Eurasian swine influenza viruses; the viruses from the initial two Californian cases were also noted to be resistant to amantadine and rimantadine, two common influenza antiviral drugs. No contact with pigs was found for any of the seven Californian nor either of the two Texas cases, suggesting human-to-human transmission of the virus.

On April 28, 2009, the director of the Centres for Disease Control and Prevention confirmed the first official US death of swine flu. Tests confirmed that a 23-month-old toddler from Mexico, who was probably infected there, died on April 27 from the flu while visiting Texas.

Outbreak Across the US

Cases of H1N1 spread rapidly across the United States, with particularly severe outbreaks in Texas, New York, and

California. Early cases were associated with recent travel to Mexico, many were students who had travelled to Mexico for Spring Break. As of May 4, 2009, the CDC reported one death, 286 confirmed cases of H1N1 flu across 36 states, 35 hospitalisations, and expects H1N1 to eventually spread to all states. A large number of cases, according to medics, have happened in the days that preceded the launch of the alert and came out only in these days due to a massive backlog. By May 5, 2009, the number has risen to 403 and a second death was reported in Texas, although it's not clear the flu was the cause of her death. The CDC and government officials have recently expressed cautious optimism about the severity and spread of H1N1.

Changes in surveillance of cases of influenza-like illness, including new guidelines for identifying cases to test, increased laboratory testing, and new test kits able to distinguish this novel strain, resulted in a spike in the per cent of cases tested that were positive for influenza. Of the positive cases, about a third were due to the novel strain. Also found were a substantial number of cases where the strain could not be subtyped. Some have claimed that illegal immigrants were significantly contributing to the spread of the swine flu.

2009 US Swine Flu Summary

Number of Confirmed Cases/Deaths	60
Number of States/Territories with Confirmed Cases	50
Earliest Confirmed Infection in US	March 28, 2009
First Death Inside the US	April 27, 2009
First Death of US Citizen	May 5, 2009
Number of People Hospitalised	770 (as of June 4)

Flu Strain Severity

The new strain was identified as a combination of several different strains of Influenzavirus A, subtype H1N1, including separate strains of this subtype circulating in humans and in pigs. The strain transmits between humans and has been reported to have a relatively high mortality rate in Mexico. The World Health Organisation (WHO) and the US Centres for Disease Control and Prevention (CDC) have expressed serious concerns that the new strain has the potential to become an influenza pandemic. It is reported that, because the virus is already widespread, containment will be impossible.

In addition, the flu death toll in Mexico could be lower than first thought, Dr. Gregory Evans, head of the Association of Medical Microbiology and Infectious Disease Canada and a member of a federal pandemic-planning committee, said on April 29:

There was a lot of speculation and what seemed to be evidence there were dozens and dozens of deaths. Careful analysis showed these people likely died of something else, and not influenza. That's really good news, and that would fit with what we've seen outside of Mexico.

Moreover, another Canadian expert, Dr. Neil Rau, criticised the WHO's decision to raise its Pandemic alert to level 5, saying:

I don't agree with (the WHO) because I think it's a panic metre, not a pandemic metre. [...] If that flu-like illness is not deadly, I don't know what the cause for alarm is for people who are not really sickened by this virus. [...] I'm really eager to know how much worse this is than seasonal flu. So far it's looking like it's not that serious.

In comparison, CNN stated on April 28, 2009 that there were at least 800 deaths in the US due to normal influenza in each individual week between January 1 and April 18, which is higher than the combined worldwide death toll for the swine flu.

However, the strain could be classified as severe due to the rapid rise in deaths over the past couple of days.

Response: The Federal response remains at US Pandemic Stage 0, congruent with the World Health Organisation (WHO) Pandemic Phases 1, 2 and 3; however, the WHO's Pandemic

Phase was raised to 4 on April 27, which is congruent with US Pandemic Stage 2. On April 29, the WHO raised the pandemic alert level to phase 5.

The United States federal government declared a public health emergency, and several US states have indicated they may follow suit. Secretary of Homeland Security Janet Napolitano noted that this declaration was standard operating procedure, which was also done for the 2009 presidential inauguration and for flooding.

White House: An official for the White House said on April 24 that "the White House is taking the situation seriously and monitoring for any new developments. The president has been fully briefed." President Barack Obama stated that "We are closely monitoring the emerging cases of swine flu". He also noted, "This is obviously a cause for concern ... but it is not a cause for alarm". President Obama suggested US schools should consider shutting down as a future possibility if students are infected. White House Press Secretary, Robert Gibbs said the effort to get a team in place to respond to the health scare has not been hindered by the lack of a secretary of Health and Human Services or appointees in any of the department's 19 key posts. The president's nominee, Kansas Gov. Kathleen Sebelius, was still awaiting confirmation from the US Senate until passing on April 28. The President has not yet made appointments to either the Commissioner of the Food and Drug Administration, the Surgeon General, or the Director of the Centres for Disease Control and Prevention. The current acting Surgeon General, Steven K. Galson, is also currently serving as the Acting Assistant Secretary for Health.

On April 30, it was reported that an aide to Steven Chu, the US Energy Secretary, had fallen ill from the virus after helping arrange President Barack Obama's trip to Mexico. However, the White House stated that the President is not at risk of obtaining the flu. Kathleen Sebelius was confirmed as the Secretary of Health and Human Services by the Senate on April 28, 2009 with a vote of 65-31.

Centres for Disease Control and Prevention (CDC)

Activation of Emergency Operations Centre During the week of April 19, the CDC activated its Emergency Operations Centre (EOC) to augment the ongoing investigation of human cases of swine influenza A (H1N1). More than 250 CDC professionals are working from the CDC EOC as part of the agency's response. As of May 4, 2009, the CDC reported that it had deployed 25 per cent of the supplies and medicines in the Strategic National Stockpile to the various states.

Swine Flu Test Kits As of April 29, only the CDC could confirm US swine flu cases. Dr. Besser stated during an April 30 press briefing that California and New York had diagnostic test kits, and that the kits would be sent to all states starting the following day. On May 6, the CDC announced that testing kits were now available for all states. This is expected to generate an increase in the number of confirmed cases as more states begin doing their own tests.

Influenza Reporting Requirements In the United States, the majority of the 70 National Respiratory and Enteric Virus Surveillance System (NREVSS) laboratories do not report the influenza A subtype. However, in 2007 human infection with a novel influenzavirus A became a nationally notifiable condition. Novel influenza A virus infections include all human infections with influenza A viruses that are different from currently circulating human influenza H1 and H3 viruses. These viruses include those that are subtyped as non-human in origin and those that are unsubtypable with standard methods and reagents. The new strain responsible for this outbreak was one such virus.

CDC Recommendations for Schools Initially the CDC had issued a recommendation that schools close for as long as two weeks if a student catches swine flu. Some school districts closed all schools if a single child was classified as probable. On May 5 the CDC retracted its advice stating that schools that were closed based on previous CDC guidance related to this outbreak may reopen. By that time at least 726 schools nationwide serving more than 480,000 students had closed for at least some period of time. The CDC amended its advice citing, new information on disease severity and the limiting effectiveness of school closure as a control measure. The new advice given stated, "Decisions about school closure should be at the discretion of local authorities based on local considerations, including public concern and the impact of school absenteeism and staffing shortages."

Food and Drug Administration

The Food and Drug Administration (FDA) authorised emergency use of medicines and diagnostic tests for flu. (FDA is part of Department of Health and Human Services.) The FDA stated it is also responding to this threat by:

- working with other government agencies and manufacturers on a series of issues related to antiviral medications.
- growing the 2009 H1N1 flu virus and preparing to make vaccine seed lots, which may be used eventually to produce a safe and effective vaccine.
- helping to prepare reagents needed for vaccine production and coordinating closely with other public health agencies for clinical development and testing.
- accelerating access to new diagnostic tools for this 2009 H1N1 flu virus.

On May 6, 2009, the FDA announced that it had approved a new manufacturing facility for seasonal flu vaccine, owned by Sanofi Pasteur, which could also be used for manufacturing a vaccine for the new H1N1 flu strain. The FDA also issued a warning for consumers to be wary of products claiming to cure or prevent swine flu.

Other Federal Agencies

Department of Homeland Security Secretary Napolitano stated that DHS is the principal federal office for incidents such as the current H1N1 flu outbreak, and "Under that role, we have been leading a true collaborative effort." The Department of Homeland Security has a document, dated Nov. 1, 2005, entitled "National Strategy for Pandemic Influenza", detailing planning for potential pandemics.

State Department The State Department suggested travellers to Mexico stay alert and comply with guidance from Mexican public health officials, but did not impose any travel restrictions on US citizens to Mexico. However, the State Department did recommend US citizens avoid non-essential travel to Mexico.

Department of Agriculture The Department of Agriculture (USDA) reported no swine in the US have been infected so far, but the USDA is monitoring swine across the US for signs of infection.

Department of Commerce The Department of Commerce sent a letter to Russia and China requesting that those countries lift their ban on American pork products.

Department of Defence The Department of Defence (DOD) is monitoring the swine flu situation and has contingency plans to deal with such outbreaks. As of May 7, 2009, the DOD reports 104 confirmed cases among Armed Forces personnel and their families. DOD maintains daily summary and map.

Department of Education The Department of Education is providing guidance to schools in the US affected by swine flu, as well as precautions to take.

State and Local: Schools closed in many states in response to local flu outbreaks. By April 30, 2009, 300 US schools and school districts had announced closures in response to the outbreak, giving 169,000 students time off. On May 4, 2009, about 533 schools in 24 states in the US were closed, affecting about 330,000 students.

On May 5, Kathleen Sebelius stated in a CDC news conference that school closures for single confirmed cases of H1N1 influenza were unnecessary, but that parents keep their child home if he or she displays an influenza-like illness.

Travel Industry

Several airlines are waiving fees for cancellations and flight changes. At least one cruise line changed itinerary to avoid Mexican ports of call.

Affected States

Alabama: On May 2, 2009, the Alabama Department of Public Health confirmed the first case of H1N1 (swine flu) in Madison, Alabama, one of two probable cases previously identified at an elementary school in Madison. As a result, all public schools and most private schools and daycare centres in Madison County, Alabama, including the cities of Huntsville and Madison, closed for two days. After meeting with the state public health officer on May 3, 2009, all Madison city elementary schools were to be closed through May 13, 2009, but were reopened after the CDC updated its guidance to schools.

As of May 8, 2009, the Alabama Department of Public Health reports 4 confirmed and 27 probable cases of swine flu.

Alaska: On May 10, 2009, the Alaska state Division of Public Health reported the state's first probable case of swine flu in a crew member of a Royal Caribbean cruise ship travelling in Alaska waters. On May 12, they confirmed that the individual had been infected with swine flu but they do not consider it to be Alaska's first case because she became ill before entering state waters.

Arizona: As of June 1, the CDC has reported a total of 547 confirmed cases and 4 deaths in the state of Arizona. The Arizona Department of Health Services reported a total of 553 confirmed cases in 14 of the state's 15 counties, with 4 deaths attributed to the illness. To date, deaths have been reported in Maricopa, Pima and Pinal counties, the state's most populous counties. Rural Greenlee County is the last county to remain free of reported human cases of the virus.

On April 28, Arizona's Department of Health submitted samples from four patients to the CDC for testing. Those four samples were confirmed to be H1N1 swine flu virus, and were all from elementary-school students in the Phoenix metropolitan area. Following recommendations from the CDC, local health authorities ordered the 3 area schools where the students attended to be closed for a period of 7 days beginning on May 1. After only 3 days, however, the order was rescinded and the schools reopened ahead of schedule on May 5 when it appeared the H1N1 flu would be no more deadly than the seasonal flu.

State health officials informed that they had 58, 000 antiviral treatment courses on hand, and that they had received over 200, 000 doses from the Strategic National Stockpile.

The first death in the state due to H1N1 swine flu complications was reported by the Maricopa County Department of Public Health on May 14. The woman, in her late-40s, had died the previous week at an undisclosed location in the county. The report indicated that the woman had suffered from an underlying respiratory ailment but did not elaborate on her condition. Subsequent victims were a 57-year-old resident of the Gila River Indian Community, a 13-year-old boy from Tucson and a pre-teen girl from Pima County.

Arkansas: As of May 8, 2009, the Arkansas Department of Health reported 5 confirmed cases of swine flu. Four of the cases were from Camp Robinson, a US Army National Guard base located in North Little Rock in Pulaski County.

California: The first two cases detected in the US were two children living in San Diego County and Imperial County (a county in which 18 per cent of their residents are not US citizens), who became ill on March 28 and 30 respectively. A CDC alert concerning these two isolated cases was reported in the media on April 21. As of April 24 eight human cases were known in the US, including six in Southern California. The patients have recovered. The acting director of the US Centres for Disease Control (CDC) said that preliminary tests on seven out of fourteen samples from patients in Mexico had matched the virus found in the US, which experts say is a new strain of swine flu. None of the US patients had any contact with pigs, leading CDC officials to believe that human-to-human transmission has been occurring.

Gov. Arnold Schwarzenegger and the state of California activated the Joint Emergency Operations Centre of the Department of Public Health, and are coordinating with the California Emergency Management Agency, the CDC, and the Mexican government. They have additionally stepped up other preparations to lessen the flu's threat. On April 28, Gov. Schwarzenegger declared a state of emergency which allows the state to deploy additional resources to the Department of Public Health and more quickly and easily purchase equipment and materials.

St. Mels Catholic School in Fair Oaks was closed after Sacramento County Health Department notified the school that a 7th grade student who reportedly recently returned from a family vacation in Mexico tested positive for an unidentified strain of Influenzavirus A. On April 27, CDC officials confirmed that the student tested positive for swine flu. In Marin County, a grandmother and her 20-month-old granddaughter have been confirmed to have the flu. By April 28, the CDC had confirmed 10 cases of swine flu in California.

California State University, Long Beach reported on April 29 that a student had returned a "probable positive" test result for swine influenza. The student showed symptoms on Sunday April 26 and went to the campus health services office the following day. The test results were received by the school on April 28 and distributed to all students and faculty. The affected student had not attended any classes since falling ill and has an apparently mild case of the disease that does not appear life threatening. Three high schools in Riverside County were closed April 29 after two teenage girls, from Corona and Indio respectively, were confirmed to have contracted the virus. Branham High School in San Jose was closed that day for a week after one teenage girl was confirmed to be a probable case. Rucker Elementary School in Gilroy is set to be closed on Friday, May 1 after at least one student was being tested after exhibiting flu-like symptoms. Three students at the Grizzly Youth Academy in San Luis Obispo are confirmed cases of swine influenza. As many as 73 students are exhibiting flu-like symptoms at The Academy and are assumed to have the virus. All are being isolated. The Academy is set to stay open. More recently, on May 3, 2009, parent of students attending King Middle School in Berkeley were notified that their school would be closed down due to a swine flu outbreak involving students at the school.

On June 1, 2009, the first two deaths were confirmed, one by a middle aged man in San Bernardino County, and another one by a middle-aged woman in Los Angeles County. A third death was confirmed on June 4, when a child from Contra Costa County died. As of June 4, there are 576 confirmed cases, 266 probable cases, and 3 deaths caused by the H1N1 flu.

Colorado: On April 30 two cases of the flu virus were confirmed in the state of Colorado. The confirmed cases were a woman from Arapahoe County who recently returned from a cruise to Mexico and a Denver International Airport baggage handler. Two more were confirmed on May 2, both in Jefferson County, Colorado. One case is a middle school student, which has caused his school to close for a week. The tally increased to seven on May 4 when The University of Colorado at Boulder (CU) confirmed three of its students contracted the virus.

Connecticut: On April 28, it was announced that there were suspected cases of swine flu in three Connecticut towns. Schools were closed due to suspected cases in East Haddam and Wethersfield, though tests on these patients later came back negative. On April 30, two students at Fairfield University were announced as having "probable" swine flu, in addition to another person in Glastonbury, bringing the total number of likely cases to 6. On May 1, the first confirmed case of swine flu was reported in Connecticut in Stratford. On May 2, the second confirmed case was reported in a child from Middlefield that had recently returned from a family trip to Mexico. On May 5, Fairfield University announced that two "probable" cases had tested positive for the H1N1 flu, with five other "probable" cases awaiting test results. One May 8, Fairfield announced that those five students had also tested positive, although the students by that time were nearly recovered, and there remained one "probable" case remained to be confirmed. On Wednesday, June 3, The first death confirmed to be linked to the H1N1 virus happened in New Haven County

Delaware: The first probable cases of swine flu in Delaware were reported on Monday, April 27. Four probable cases of swine flu were reported on the University of Delaware campus after the students were experiencing flu like symptoms. Tests were sent to the CDC to see if the students had the swine flu. All four cases were confirmed by the CDC on April 28. The students were reported to be recovering, and the campus set up a temporary Public Health clinic. The Delaware Division of Public Health reported on May 1 a further 17 probable cases, all from the University.

District of Columbia: As of May 10, 2009, the DC Department of Health reported 4 confirmed and 6 probable cases of swine flu.

Florida: On April 28, it was reported that an individual in Florida had tested positive for influenza type A, of which swine flu is a subtype. A culture from that person has been sent to Jacksonville to be tested for swine flu, with results expected within 48 hours. Governor Crist announced the first two confirmed cases in Florida on May 1. The cases are both children and in Lee and Broward counties.

On May 3, the Hillsborough County Health Department announced 5 possible cases of H1N1, 4 of the persons are students, and the other is a relative who has recently travelled to Mexico. Three public schools (Wilson Middle School, Freedom High School, and Liberty Middle School) where the students attended have been closed till May 11.

On May 7, Alachua County announced its first case of H1N1 (Swine Flu). The person is a University of Florida student and has since recovered.

On May 8, a 7-year-old boy tested positive of swine influenza in Rockledge, Brevard County, Florida . Two other children tested positive for influenza. It caused Golfview Elementary School in Rockledge to close on May 11.

Georgia: The first case of laboratory confirmed swine flu was reported on April 30. A Kentucky woman was hospitalised in LaGrange while visiting family in Georgia; she had recently returned from a trip to Mexico. While Georgia health officials reported this as a confirmed case for the state, the CDC and the Kentucky health department reported it as a case in Kentucky. In relation to this case, state officials said they had no plans to close schools or other public institutions.

On May 4, the Georgia Department of Human Resources announced that all classes have been temporarily suspended at Eagle's Landing Christian Academy in Henry County until the CDC confirms the status of a student who became ill. The Georgia Public Health Laboratory sent three probable cases to the CDC over the weekend for confirmation. On May 5, the Georgia Division of Public Health confirmed three cases of H1N1 located in Cobb, DeKalb and Henry Counties.

Hawaii: On May 4, 2009, the Hawaii Department of Health announced that there were three suspected cases of swine flu in the state. Governor Linda Lingle announced that the cases were mild and that the patients were recovering at home. On May 5, 2009, all three cases were confirmed on the island of Oahu by the CDC. All three cases involve recent travel to the mainland United States. One case is a school-age child, who recently travelled to California. The two other cases are a military member, and his or her spouse. The military member travelled to Texas, and has exposed their spouse.

Two more cases were confirmed on May 6. Another four were confirmed on May 13, with two identified at Anuenue School, a Hawaiian language immersion school. In response to the outbreak, the University of Hawaii at Manoa announced that it will not be shaking graduates' hands at its commencement.

Idaho: On Sunday, May 3, 2009, The Centres for Disease Control and Prevention confirmed the state's first swine flu infection for a Kootenai County woman in her 60s. As of Tuesday, May 6, 2009, an infant from Ada County was being tested for a probable case.

Illinois: The state's first probable case of swine flu was reported on Wednesday, April 29. An elementary school in Chicago's Rogers Park neighbourhood, on the city's Far North Side, was closed because a 12-year-old student was presumed to have the disease. The student reportedly was recovering at home. By April 30, over 40 probable cases had been identified by state and local health officials. In addition to 16 cases in the city of Chicago, and 11 in surrounding Cook County, cases were reported in Kane, Lake, DuPage, McHenry, and Will counties. Several schools in the affected areas were temporarily closed. Many other flu cases happened during or even before the launch of the alert were then confirmed, principally in the urban area of Chicago. By May 20, the following 17 counties had confirmed cases: Boone, Cook, DeKalb, DuPage, Franklin, Kane, Kankakee, Kendall, Knox, Lake, McDonough, McHenry, Ogle, Sangamon, Will, Williamson, and Winnebago. Total confirmed cases in Illinois were 794, up from 707 the previous day.

Cases in Illinois throughout May 2009 continued to climb and by May 31, 2009 the published CDC numbers had reached 1002 confirmed cases with 2 deaths. A third confirmed death — the first outside of the Chicago metropolitan area — was reported by state health authorities on May 28, 2009 but this was not reflected in the CDC official numbers by the end of the month.

Indiana: On April 28, an unidentified Notre Dame student was confirmed as the first case of swine flu in this state. The patient had not recently travelled to Mexico or been in contact with anyone who has travelled to Mexico. The student was in voluntarily quarantine, and was doing well, according to Judy Monroe, Indiana's state health commissioner. Two other cases in the state which occurred in two Indianapolis elementary schools were confirmed by the CDC shortly thereafter. Additional cases later surfaced in the counties of Hendricks, Lake, Marion, Putnam, St. Joseph, and Tippecanoe.

Iowa: On April 29, two probable case of swine flu were reported in Des Moines County and Clinton County. One was a woman from California, the other one was a man from Mexico. On May 3, another case was found in Marshall County causing schools to close. On the week of February 28, 2009, a three-year old caught the swine flu due to close contact with ill pigs, but not the same dangerous strain that came from Mexico. In early-May, cases climbed up to 43. A few were in Polk County, where Des Moines is.

Kansas: Health officials in Kansas announced April 25 that two new cases of swine flu had been confirmed in Dickinson County, after both were isolated. The week prior, one patient had travelled to Mexico by plane to attend a professional conference; both he and his wife experienced minor influenza symptoms.

Kentucky: A Warren County woman who had recently visited Mexico tested positive for the virus April 30. After returning to Kentucky from Mexico, she travelled to Georgia where she was hospitalised. Health officials from both states announced this as the first confirmed case in their states, however the CDC listed the case in Kentucky.

In Jefferson County, Meyzeek Middle school has three cases of H1N1 Influenza. This initially started from a staff member, but spread to students.

Counties in Kentucky with confirmed cases of the H1N1 flu:

- Boone- 2^+
- Boyle- 1
- Daviess- 1
- Fayette- 4
- Hardin- 1

- Jefferson- 26
- Kenton- 2[+]
- Lincoln- 1
- Madison- 8
- Mercer- 4
- Oldham- 1
- Scott- 7
- Warren- 1[*]

Total- 59:

[+] — *One of these cases are confirmed by a local health department.*

— *Resident of that county, but hospitalised in Georgia.*

Confirmation by various health departments:

- Centres for Disease Control and Prevention- 50
- Kentucky State Public Health Laboratory- 57
- Northern Kentucky Independent Health Department- 2

Louisiana: On May 29, there are a total of 125 swine flu cases confirmed by The Louisiana Department of Health and Hospitals. Up from 114 reported on May 28.

According to the Louisiana Department of Health and Hospitals, the confirmed cases are broken down by parish as follows:

- 3 Ascension
- 14 East Baton Rouge
- 2 Evangeline
- 3 Iberia
- 56 Lafayette
- 3 Lafourche
- 3 LaSalle
- 1 Orleans

- 12 Plaquemines
- 5 St. Charles
- 2 St. Landry
- 2 St. Martin
- 1 St. Tammany
- 1 Tangipahoa
- 2 Terrebonne
- 3 Vermillion
- 1 Vernon

Maine: On April 29 three cases of H1N1 (swine flu) were confirmed in Maine, according to the Maine Centre for Disease Control. The three adults, two from Kennebec County and one from York County, were reported to be recovering at home. Dr. Dora Anne Mills, director of Maine's CDC, said on April 28 that at least 12 suspected cases were being tested.

Late on April 29, Maine Governor John Baldacci declared a "civil emergency" and ordered a school and daycare facility in York County to close for 7 days.

Maryland: By May 1, 2009, eleven probable cases had been identified in Maryland, in Anne Arundel, Baltimore, Charles, Prince Georges, and Montgomery Counties. One of these cases, that of a high school student in Rockville, resulted in the closing of Rockville High School, the first Maryland school closing due to the outbreak. On May 1, three other schools in the state were closed. As of May 5, Rockville High School has reopened. Four of Maryland's probable cases were confirmed on May 4, including two adults and one child in Baltimore County as well as one young child in Anne Arundel county.

Massachusetts: There are 854 confirmed cases in Massachusetts, 6.7 per cent of which have led to hospitalisations. Confirmed cases by county

- 7 Barnstable
- 2 Berkshire

- 10 Bristol
- 34 Essex
- 1 Franklin
- 2 Hampden
- 6 Hampshire
- 287 Middlesex
- 1 Nantucket
- 98 Norfolk
- 16 Plymouth
- 342 Suffolk
- 48 Worcester

By County:

- *Barnstable County*
  - — A member of the US Coast Guard stationed on Cape Cod, acquired the virus while training in California, but reportedly recovered.
- *Bristol County*
  - — The Health Agent for the town of Easton stated that there are "a couple of suspected cases in town."
  - — The Mass. Dept. of Public Health announced that they had 1 confirmed case of the virus in the city of Fall River in southeastern Massachusetts.
- *Franklin County*
  - — There is at least 1 confirmed case reported in the county.
- *Hampshire County*
  - — Two students at Amherst College in Amherst had confirmed cases of the virus and 13 other students are 'suspected' cases. All 15 students are being isolated on campus. A third student at the school contracted the H1N1 virus. Also, there has been 1

'suspected' case each at Mount Holyoke College (in South Hadley) and Smith College (in Northampton).

- *Middlesex County*
  - — The Massachusetts Department of Public Health informed the Ashland school superintendent that two Ashland High School students have "probable" cases of H1N1 flu.
  - — The CDC confirmed that an elementary school student in Chelmsford tested positive for acquiring the virus.
  - — In Cambridge, there are 2 students (at the Massachusetts Institute of Technology) that are "probable" cases of having acquired the virus.
  - — Eight residents of Framingham are being tested for being "probable" cases.
  - — The Lincoln Public Schools Superintendent had confirmed a Lincoln middle school student been diagnosed with the H1N1 virus.
  - — Two middle school students in Lowell have tested positive for swine flu as of April 29, 2009. The two had gone on a family trip to Mexico, and became mildly sick on returning home. The local health department said that the boys had not returned to school since coming back from Mexico, and there were no concerns that the illness had been spread.
  - — In Tyngsboro, there had been 1 probable case reported at the Academy of Notre Dame.
  - — There is 1 suspected case of the virus in the city of Waltham.
  - — Winchester Hospital in Winchester reported having received a possible case (of the virus) within the town.
  - — There had been two additional confirmed cases, 1 of each located in the municipalities of Bedford and Weston.

— In Wayland there has been one confirmed case at the elementary school level and one possible case at the high school level.

- *Norfolk County*

— The health inspector of Quincy confirmed that a New York resident who checked into Quincy Medical Centre on May 1, 2009, and tested positive for the H1N1 flu.

— The CDC confirmed that a resident of the Wellesley College campus tested positive for the virus.

— The Dana Hall School in Wellesley was closed after nearly 100 students called in sick.

- *Plymouth County*

— The CDC had announced 4 additional confirmed cases, from 2 adults and 2 school-age residents (of the state), from the following counties: (3) Middlesex County and (1) Plymouth County.

- *Suffolk County*

— Massachusetts' Secretary of Health and Human Services announced that 'some' of the 34 confirmed cases in the state are from the Harvard School of Dental Medicine campus (at the Longwood Medical Area in Boston), which is temporarily closed. Later, it was reported that 3 of the 9 reported cases of influenza at the school, resulted positive for the H1N1 virus.

— On May 1, 2009, a United Airlines Flight 903 from Munich to Washington D.C., was diverted to Logan International Airport in Boston. A 53-year-old passenger complained of flu-like symptoms, that led him to be admitted to Massachusetts General Hospital.

— A male passenger in his 40s complained of flu-like symptoms upon landing at Logan International

Airport in Boston May 2, 2009. He was flying aboard American Airlines Flight 155, from London to Boston, that had originated from Malaysia. He, too, was admitted to Massachusetts General Hospital in Boston.

— The Boston University Goldman School of Dental Medicine reported a single resident that has a confirmed case of the virus. They claim that he has had no contact with anybody on the school's main campus, and those he has been in contact with have been notified.

— Both Boston Latin, where 250 called in sick, and the Winsor School, where 34 called in sick, and were closed.

- *Worcester County*

— There is at least 1 confirmed case reported in the county.

- *Other*

— In Spencer, two students who also had recently returned from Mexico were tested for possible swine flu infection. The results of those tests were both negative.

Michigan: On April 29, a 34-year-old woman from Livingston County was Michigan's first reported case of swine flu. On April 30, another 34-year-old woman from Ottawa County was confirmed as Michigan's second case. As of June 2, Michigan reports 298 confirmed flu cases, and one death.

The death in Michigan was of a 53-year-old women who lived in Warren, Michigan and had other underlying health problems.

Confirmed cases by county:

- 2 Allegan
- 2 Bay
- 5 Berrien
- 1 Branch

- 4 Calhoun
- 2 Chippewa
- 1 Clare
- 1 Clinton
- 2 Eaton
- 6 Genessee
- 1 Hillsdale
- 3 Ingham
- 1 Ionia
- 2 Isabella
- 8 Kalamazoo
- 51 Kent
- 15 Livingston
- 20 Macomb
- 5 Missaukee
- 8 Monroe
- 2 Montcalm
- 3 Muskegon
- 1 Newaygo
- 68 Oakland
- 1 Oceana
- 16 Ottawa
- 1 Roscommon
- 1 Saginaw
- 1 St. Clair
- 3 Van Buren
- 26 Washtenaw
- 34 Wayne

Minnesota: On April 30, 2009, the Minnesota Department of Health announced that the first case of "H1N1 novel influenza virus" in the state was confirmed by the CDC. The infected individual is an unidentified resident of Cold Spring, Minnesota. Two schools in the affected city will remain closed until May 6, 2009.

On May 4, 2009 the second case of H1N1 was confirmed in Minnesota by the Minnesota Department of Health. The case was reported in a teen boy attending a Minneapolis Public School. As of May 6, 2009 three more cases of swine flu are suspected in kids attending multiple Minneapolis Public Schools.

Another case of H1N1 was confirmed in a worker who was taking pigs to Texas and brought it back up to the small town of Mountain Lake.

Mississippi: On May 15, 2009 Mississippi State officials reported three cases in Harrison County, Mississippi. As of May 28, 2009, Mississippi State officials reported 20 cases in the state in 4 counties in the south towards the coast. The other county in the north. 4 days later it spread further with now 34 cases.

Forrest County: 2 Lamar County: 4 Union County: 1 Jackson County: 10 Harrison County: 11 Desoto County: 1 Holmes County: 1 Yazoo County: 2.

Missouri: In Missouri, Gov. Jay Nixon announced in a written statement that a probable case had been discovered in a Platte County man, and that a sample had been sent to the CDC for confirmation.

As of May 8, 2009, the Missouri Department of Health and Senior Services (DHSS) reported 10 confirmed and 4 probable cases of swine flu.

On May 19, 2009, a St. Louis County man became the first death in Missouri due to the Swine Flu.

On May 21, 2009, St. Louis Public School District announced one of its students had the Swine Flu but has not been in class since May 15.

In St. Charles Missouri it was also found that a student from St. Charles High School who travelled to Mexico City was found infected with swine flu. Eric Trejo the student who just came back from Mexico City was in school for a week than kicked out and brought back.

Montana: As of May 11, 2009, the Montana Department of Public Health and Human Services (DPHHH) reported the state's first confirmed case of swine flu.

Nebraska: There are 29 confirmed cases of swine flu in Nebraska, with six probable cases.

Nevada: The first confirmed case of the virus was reported in Nevada on April 29. A two year-old girl from Reno contracted the virus, but it is unclear how as the case did not appear to be linked to any previously affected areas. As of recent the virus has spread to Clark County, where the city of Las Vegas lies. It has also resulted in the closing of Mendive Middle

School in Sparks, Reno's neighbouring city, where ten students were confirmed to have contracted the virus.

New Hampshire: The New Hampshire Department of Health and Human Services announced the state's first confirmed case of the H1N1 flu May 2, 2009. The confirmed case involves an employee of Concord Hospital in Concord, New Hampshire.

New Jersey: As of May 29, 2009, the New Jersey Government has confirmed 75 cases of swine flu and 6 probable cases, most of them within a range of 30 minutes of New York or Philadelphia. More swine flu cases are being reported daily, which has caused a widespread in the state. Counties currently confirmed with swine flu: Bergen (7), Burlington (8), Camden (8), Essex (5), Hudson (12), Mercer (5), Middlesex (3), Monmouth (11), Morris (7), Ocean (2), Passaic (2), Somerset (1), Sussex (1), Union (1), Warren (2), which indicates that currently 15 counties have confirmed cases of swine flu.

New Mexico: On April 29, 2009, Gov. Bill Richardson announced that there are two very probable cases in New Mexico. The suspected cases were a 1-year-old boy from Santa Fe County and an 18-year-old man from Valencia County. The 1-year old tested negative for H1N1, but the 18-year-old man tested positive. More cases were raised in the intervening days, and by May 1 the probable case number was increased to nine. In addition to the cases above, a 17-year-old girl from Eddy County, a 22-year-old woman also from Eddy County, a 15-year-old girl from Valencia County, a 17-year-old boy from Hidalgo County, and a 27-year-old man from Bernalillo County are also likely to be infected.

As of May 19, 2009 the New Mexico Department of Health has confirmed 76 total cases of the H1N1 virus among humans in various counties. 8 new were confirmed on May 19 itself.

New York: On April 24, New York City Department of Health and Mental Hygiene dispatched a team of investigators to the private St. Francis Preparatory School in Queens after

150 students complained of symptoms consistent with the disease. Several of the students had recently travelled to Mexico City..New York City Health Commissioner Dr. Thomas Frieden reported on April 25 that eight of the New York school cases were "probable" swine flu.

On April 26 the Centres for Disease Control and Prevention (CDC) confirmed that the Queens cases are indeed associated with the H1N1 virus. The students suffered only mild symptoms, and some have since recovered.

On April 27 federal officials confirmed 20 new US cases at the same school in New York in which eight cases were confirmed earlier.

As of April 29, one undergraduate commuter student on the Queens Campus of St. John's University had contracted the Swine Flu (A/H1N1) virus. The student was treated and recovered.

On May 14, three New York City public schools were closed due to the flu symptoms of hundreds of students.

On May 17, Mitchell Wiener, the assistant principal at a Queens school was confirmed as New York State's first death due to the disease.

On May 24, a woman in her 50s died because of the disease and had other health problems. She is New York State's second death and the 11th in the country. On June 1st a child from the Bronx became the first minor in New York City to die of swine flu. On Wednesday, June 4th, a man died in Onondaga County, which marked the first fatality from swine flu in New York outside of New York City.

As of June 4, there are 866 confirmed cases of the H1N1 flu.

North Carolina: The state health director, Dr. Jeffrey Engel, announced that there had been two probable cases of swine flu in the state. The first case was a man travelling through Wake County, where the capital is located, on business. The other case was an Onslow County resident who had recently travelled to Texas. On a related note, North Carolina is one of

29 states that have deemed to have not stockpiled enough flu medicines by federal guidelines. However, Dr. Engel dismissed these concerns, saying, "I think the commercial supply will keep up at the present time."

Ohio: On April 26, the Ohio Department of Health reported that a nine-year-old boy attending Elyria City Schools in Elyria, Lorain County, had been diagnosed with a mild case of the new strain of swine influenza and that his immediate family was undergoing testing. After the confirmed case in Ohio and eight in New York occurred Federal officials declared a public health emergency. The Cleveland health department received numerous calls from concerned residents the first week of the outbreak, although it has been difficult to tell whether or not the cases are swine flu, since it is regular flu season. On April 29, a probable case was reported in Columbus, and two new cases were confirmed in Columbus on May 2, one of them being an employee of The Ohio State University Medical Centre.

Oklahoma: In Muskogee, Oklahoma a man who recently visited Mexico had been admitted into a hospital after having H1N1 flu symptoms, but test results on May 1 returned negative. On May 5, a woman from Pontotoc County was confirmed to have H1N1 flu, On May 7, Oklahoma State Department of Health confirmed three new cases of the H1N1 virus: a child from Oklahoma County, and one adult and a teenage female in Cleveland County. All have recovered.

Oregon: The first probable case of H1N1 flu in Oregon was announced on April 30th by the Oregon Department of Human Services. By May 3rd, three people had been tested positive for swine flu. On May 22nd the ODHS announced that 46 per cent of patients who tested positive for flu since March 4th were indeed infected with H1N1 flu, with the rest having just a seasonal flu.

H1N1 has been detected in 159 residents of Oregon as of June 2nd, 2009. Confirmed cases have been found in 13 out of 36 counties, including Clackamas County, Clatsop County, Columbia County, Jackson County, Lane County, Lincoln

County, Linn County, Marion County, Multnomah County, Polk County, Umatilla County, Washington County, and Yamhill County.

No deaths have been reported in the State of Oregon.

Pennsylvania: On May 3, The Pennsylvania Department of Health said that a 31-year-old male in Montgomery County had the H1N1 flu. Another resident from Montgomery County was also confirmed to have the virus on May 5. There are also confirmed cases in the following counties: Allegheny (1), Berks (16), Bucks (2), Chester (1), Luzerne (1), Lycoming (1), Montgomery (2), and Philadelphia (15). More cases are currently being tested. Several probable cases are also located in the following counties: ten in Philadelphia, two in Bucks, two in Chester, as well as one each in Allegheny, Cambria, Franklin, Lehigh, Luzerne, Lycoming, Montgomery, and York.

On June 4, a 55-year-old woman in Harrisburg was confirmed as the first death in Pennsylvania due to swine flu.

On June 7, a 27-year-old woman died of Swine flu.

Rhode Island: On May 2, 2009, Rhode Island confirmed its first case of H1N1 Flu in a Westerly woman. As of May 8, 2009, the Rhode Island Department of Health reported 7 confirmed and 1 probable case of swine flu.

South Carolina: 13 cases of the flu virus were confirmed in South Carolina on April 30. All 13 were students or parents from the private Newberry Academy in Newberry, South Carolina; many had travelled to Mexico earlier in the month. All nearby public schools were closed for May 1. The S.C. Department of Health said there were nine more probable cases, and a further 22 cases still under investigation throughout the state.

South Dakota: Test results for two suspected cases of swine flu in South Dakota came back negative. The University of Nebraska Medical Centre looked into suspicious specimens to determine if a Nebraska resident had the flu. However, the test turned up negative, but the Medical centre is currently testing more than a dozen other specimens for the strain.

Tennessee: Officials announced that in Williamson County that a child in Middle Tennessee is believed to have swine flu. The child's school, Harding Academy in Davidson County, has been closed. A second possible case of swine flu in Collierville has been reported in Tennessee. Medical tests at St. Jude Children's Research Hospital indicate the child has swine flu. Incarnation Catholic School the second child's school, has also been closed for the next week, per CDC guidelines. Another possible case has been identified in Knox County for a student who attends West Valley Middle School.

Texas: Of the first 5 deaths and 1,499 cases confirmed in Texas, one was a Mexican citizen.

Two students attending Byron P. Steele II High School in Cibolo were confirmed to have the A/H1N1 swine flu; the patients recovered. A third possible case in a student who attends the same high school as the two other cases in Texas has been identified and the school is closed temporarily. On April 25, the Texas Department of State Health Services (DSHS) decided to close Byron P. Steele II High School for the following week. Following the discovery of more possible swine flu illnesses, the DSHS ordered that all schools and district facilities in the Schertz-Cibolo-Universal City Independent School District be closed for the week.

On April 27, a 7-year-old, a 24-year-old, and a 3-month-old in Dallas County were confirmed to have swine flu. All recovering and were not hospitalised. That same day, the Richardson Independent School District in the northern Dallas suburb of Richardson shut down Canyon Creek Elementary School due to a confirmed and two suspected cases of swine flu. All schools in New Braunfels—private schools and all campuses of the Comal and New Braunfels Independent School Districts—announced closures through May 10 on the recommendation of the Medical Authority of Comal County. On May 6, the *New Braunfels Herald-Zeitung* reported that all schools in Guadalupe and Comal counties would reopen on Thursday, May 7, four days earlier than had previously been announced.

Due to the swine flu, the University Interscholastic League (UIL) suspended all athletic, musical, and academic competitions and games for primary and secondary public education in the state of Texas until May 11.

On April 28, the City of Houston Health Department and Texas Children's Hospital sent samples in to the CDC. There are also possible cases at the Baylor College of Medicine outpatient clinic, Memorial Hermann Hospital, and St. Luke's Hospital.

A 23-month-old Mexican toddler who had been brought to Houston from Brownsville died on April 27, making the child the first US death due to the outbreak. The child had travelled with his family from Mexico to Brownsville to visit relatives. The infant was admitted to a Brownsville hospital after becoming ill, then transferred to Texas Children's Hospital the next day. The toddler suffered from chronic muscle weakness, a heart defect, a swallowing problem and lack of oxygen.

Texas Governor Rick Perry issued a disaster declaration.

On April 29, it was confirmed by Harris County that a 17-year-old girl from Fort Bend County attending Episcopal High School in Bellaire had contracted and recovered from the A/H1N1 swine flu. In compliance with the directives of the Harris County Public Health and Environmental Services Department, the school has been closed until further notice. Also in Fort Worth, a rising number of possible and confirmed cases in the district made school officials close all schools starting the next day, April 30. Schools in FWISD remained closed until May 8. The district was the biggest in the nation to close resulting in 80,000 students out of school and 11,000 staff members out of their jobs for that time. During the next week 6 school districts in Dallas-Fort Worth shut down. Including Cleburne, Lewisville, Decatur, Denton, Fort Worth, and Ponder. Other schools in Plano, Dallas, and Richardson were also closed, but did not result in a district wide shut down. Other smaller districts also shut down. Also that day, a probable case caused the closure of Lucy Read Pre-Kindergarten Demonstration School in north Austin.

Denton County reported its first confirmed swine flu case April 30, in a child in Plano; the student attended Wilson Middle School in the Plano Independent School District, and the district decided to close the Collin County school until May 11. Navo Middle School and Lee Elementary School, of Denton Independent School District were also closed after three students at both schools respectively were diagnosed with type A influenza. As of May 2, the rest of Denton ISD officially closed for the following week, but as of May 5, all schools are officially reopening on May 7.

The Superintendent of Keller Independent School District in Keller reported 3 possible cases, one in each of three schools.

On April 30, 8 suspected cases were recognised in El Paso County. Lab samples have been sent to CDC. No further information has been provided at this time until cases are confirmed. At this time, international borders will remain open. The El Paso Dept. of Public Health identified 11 more suspect cases of H1N1 flu in El Paso County on Friday, May 1, to bring the total number of suspect cases to 19. Lamar Consolidated ISD closed Lamar Junior High School due to a suspected (probable) case. Weslaco ISD closed all campuses for 7 days after a student was confirmed to have contracted type A influenza.

On May 5, Judy Trunnell, a woman in her 30s suffering from "chronic underlying health conditions" died of swine flu in Cameron County, near the US-Mexico border. She was the first US citizen to die from the disease. The woman, a special education teacher, had recently given birth to an eight-month-term healthy baby, delivered by caesarian section. She had been in a coma after being admitted to the hospital with breathing problems on April 19. The woman had also suffered from asthma, rheumatoid arthritis and a skin condition.

Utah: On April 28, 2009, one student in Park City, Utah was suspected to have swine flu. Two more students in the school district began showing similar symptoms making three probable cases. All 8 schools in the Park City School District closed the following day. On May 1 the number of probable cases was increased to 9; 6 in Summit County (Park City), 2 in Salt Lake County and 1 in the Morgan-Weber Health District and about 80 suspected cases. May 2 at around 11 o'clock the first confirmation came back for the original case, 7 more were confirmed by the 6th. On May 6 the probable case count was at 30. The first confirmed death from swine flu in Utah, of a 21-year-old man, was reported on May 20, 2009.

Vermont: The Vermont Department of Health announced a probable case of the H1N1 virus in rural Orleans County. A second case of the flu was confirmed involving an adult in Windsor County.

Virginia: The Virginia Department of Health had confirmed 14 cases in the state by May 7, and a total of 23 by May 21. The VDH reports cases by Health district, often without narrowing down a specific county, citing HIPAA privacy laws, as well as a desire to avoid creating a "false sense of security". 12 of the cases have been reported for the district containing Lexington, Virginia, following an early outbreak on the campus of Washington and Lee University. Additionally, there have been three cases in Fairfax, two each in the Chesterfield, Arlington and Peninsula Health districts, and one each in the Norfolk and Three Rivers Health districts.

Washington: As of the evening of May 22, 2009, Washington state has reported 574 confirmed cases, one probable case, and one death due to Swine Flu. So far, confirmed cases have been identified in seventeen Washington state counties, with public facilities closed as a precaution in those counties and several others. On May 3, Seattle-King County officials announced that, due to the virus' widespread presence in the community and low rates of severity, schools would no longer be closing due to suspect or probable cases.

A majority of confirmed cases (384) so far have occurred in King County. 115 confirmed cases, one probable case, and one death have been reported in Snohomish County. Thirty-one confirmed cases have also been identified in Pierce County. While seven cases of swine flu have been confirmed in Clark County, bordering the city of Portland, Oregon.

Thurston County and Yakima County have reported five cases. Spokane County and Whatcom County have reported four cases each. Kitsap County and Mason County have reported three cases. Two cases have been reported in Island County and Skagit County. One case each has been reported in Douglas County, Grays Harbour County, Jefferson County, Kittitas County and Lewis County. An additional case, that of a cruise ship worker, is counted at the state level only.

On May 9, it was announced that a man from Snohomish County, in his thirties with a pre-existing heart condition and active viral pneumonia, became the third confirmed US death from Swine Flu-involved complications.

Wisconsin: As of May 22, 2009, Wisconsin has 1130 confirmed cases, most of which are in the southern and southeastern region of the state. So far, cases have been confirmed in 24 counties, however Milwaukee, Dane, Waukesha, and Columbia have the majority of the cases, with 706, 90, 54, and 52 respectively. As of May 24, 2009, Wisconsin currently has the most confirmed cases of swine flu in the United States. On June 1st, 2009, it was confirmed that a Milwaukee resident with underlying health issues died from the virus.

Wyoming: As of June 4, there have been 25 confirmed cases of swine flu in Wyoming.

2009 Swine Flu Outbreak Actions Concerning Pigs

Following the 2009 swine flu outbreak, governments around the world have responded with sometimes extreme reactions against pigs, which has included the official extermination of all domestic pigs in Egypt and the culling of three wild boars at the Baghdad Zoo in Iraq. Many of these slaughters occurred in Muslim countries, and religious restrictions on the consumption of pork have been cited as influencing the decision to take such action.

The World Health Organisation (WHO) has stated that there is no reason to believe that pigs are transmitting the flu to humans.

Egypt: On 29 April 2009, the Egyptian Government announced the decision to slaughter all pigs in the country, roughly 300,000. This decision reportedly raised religious tensions since pig owners are mostly in the Coptic Christian minority in the predominantly Islamic nation. Egyptian human rights lawyer Nadia Tawfiq claimed that the pig extermination was a form of attack on Christians. Many international newspapers attributed the action to the global swine-flu outbreak even though no cases of swine flu had been reported in the country.

According to the Egyptian Ministry of Health (MOH) the extermination was not based on either the swine flu outbreak, nor it is against a specific group of citizens. On the Elkahira Elyoum TV show, Dr. Hatem El-Gabaly announced the pig extermination was based on the fear that the bird flu could mutate in the unkept pig herds. The decision was reached because so many of the areas used by pig growers are specifically trash dumps and do not follow any veterinary supervision, unlike most other countries that raise pigs in a tested and controlled environment. The extra attention and urgency by the emergence of the bird flu, then the swine flu, provided an opportunity to act on a plan that had been there for several years, . Josep Domenech, the chief veterinary officer at the UN Food and Agriculture Organisation (FAO) called the decision "a real mistake", saying that FAO had been trying to reach Egyptian officials but there has been no response.

Egypt commenced the slaughter on 2 May 2009. On the next day in Cairo, an estimated 300 Coptic Christian residents of the Manshiyat Nasr district set up blockades on the street in attempt to keep government officers from confiscating their pigs, which led to clashes with the police. *Al-Ahram*, a widely circulated Egyptian newspaper, reported that owners of destroyed pigs will receive 1000 Egyptian pounds (approximately US $177.70) per animal in compensation, but Reuters reported that the issue was still "under discussion", citing an Egyptian Cabinet spokesman.

On 10 May 2009, Islamic scholar Sheikh Ali Osman from the Egyptian Waqf ministry issued a disputed fatwa declaring that "the source of all the pigs in the world is Jews, who were cursed by Allah", and that, due to their Jewish roots, it is permissible to slaughter all the pigs. He is currently waiting for an official approval from the Al-Azhar Fatwa Committee for his new edict. There is currently a dispute between Muslim scholars about whether Jews actually come from pig. The Quran mentions that Allah cursed some of the evil people "Shall I point out to you something much worse than this, (as judged) by the treatment it received from Allah? Those who incurred the curse of Allah and His wrath, those of whom some He transformed into apes and swine, those who worshiped Evil; these are (many times) worse in rank and far more astray from the even Path!" By this reading, there is no connection between Jews and pigs, as "cursing into pigs" is meant for all evil-doers, not Jews. Egypt was also generally criticised for the brutal killing of the pigs.

Iraq: Adel Salman Musa, the director of the Baghdad Zoo claims to have "received an order issued by the multi-ministry committee aimed at preventing swine flu" to kill Baghdad's supply of three wild boars. He said the cull was initiated "to break a barrier of fear" which had been developed amongst zoo visitors. There had been a decline in the number of visitors in the days prior to the culling.

The health ministry said that killing the pigs would serve no purpose in preventing an outbreak in the country that has no reported cases of swine flu. Ehassan Jafar, a spokesperson for the country's health ministry, said that "it does not matter" since the virus is able to transmit itself between humans now. In its dispute with the agriculture ministry, the health ministry said "if you really want to kill them then just kill them".

The boars were tested prior to their culling, and results proved negative. The zoo's director said they were killed humanely. This involved the use of an anesthetic. The three carcasses were later buried.

The deaths were relayed around the world via Agence France-Presse, CNN, Israel's Ynetnews and China's Xinhua News Agency.

Iraqi Kurdistan: Kurdistan's Regional Government has outlawed boar hunting. The area has a large population of wild boars.

Inhabitants are told to avoid the consumption of pork. Travellers are being monitored for their activity in relation to this.

Afghanistan: As reported by Telegraph.co.uk, Afghanistan's only pig has been taken off display in the Kabul Zoo and "quarantined" as a response to visitor's fears.

Swine Flu Outbreak in Mexico 2009

In March and April 2009, an outbreak of a new strain of influenza commonly referred to as "swine flu" infected many people in Mexico and other parts of the world, causing illness ranging from mild to severe. Initial reports suggested that the outbreak had started in February due to farming practices at a pig farm half-owned by Smithfield Foods. Smithfield Foods stated that it had found no clinical signs or symptoms of the presence of swine influenza in the company's swine herd, or among its employees at its joint ventures in Mexico, that it routinely administers influenza virus vaccination to their swine herds and that it conducts monthly testing for the presence of swine influenza. The new strain was identified as a combination of several different strains of Influenzavirus A, subtype H1N1, including separate strains of this subtype circulating in humans and in pigs. The World Health Organisation (WHO) and the

US Centres for Disease Control and Prevention (CDC) have expressed serious concerns that the new strain, which transmits between humans and has had a relatively high mortality rate in the possible and confirmed Mexican cases, has the potential to become an influenza pandemic. It is reported that, because the virus is already widespread, containment will be impossible.

As of 27 April 2009, all schools nationwide remain closed until at least 6 May. Health Minister Cordova noted that the number of new cases had declined during the three days: from 141 on Saturday to 119 on Sunday and 110 on Monday. It is unclear why there were more deaths in Mexico than in other areas, as there were multiple potential variables, such as a stronger strain of the virus or more exposure to it. No definite conclusion had been reached, however the CDC reported that swine flu viruses in the US and Mexico matched.

Outbreak: The first infected was registered in San Diego, California on 2 April, but it was missclassed as an H2N3 case. It was not until 13 April, with the first death in Oaxaca, that further research was carried out, officially detecting the new type of virus on April 16. The pandemic outbreak was first detected in the Federal District, where surveillance began picking up a surge in cases of influenza-like illness starting on March 18. The surge was assumed by authorities to be "late-season flu" (which usually coincides with a mild Influenzavirus B peak) until April 21, when a CDC alert concerning two isolated cases of a novel swine flu was reported in the media. Both cases were in US counties on the Mexico – United States border, adjacent to one state in Mexico where the influenza surge had been detected. This was the missing link that connected the surge and the new strain, and established the high suspicion of an outbreak.

Swine Flu Outbreak in the United Kingdom 2009

The 2009 swine flu outbreak in the United Kingdom started in April 2009, involving an outbreak of a new strain of influenza commonly known as swine flu. The virus was identified as a combination of several strains of Influenzavirus A, subtype H1N1. The origins of this new strain are unknown and it has not been isolated in pigs. The virus was shown to transmit between humans leading the World Health Organisation (WHO) to be concerned about its potential to become an influenza pandemic.

The first cases were confirmed on 27 April in passengers returning from Mexico. The first case of person to person transmission within the UK was announced on 1 May.

In response to the worldwide outbreak, Foreign and Commonwealth Office advised against all but essential travel to Mexico. A number of government agencies issued guidance on what to do if anyone suspected they were infected, and the public were assured of the plans in place for an influenza pandemic.

England's chief medical officer Sir Liam Donaldson warned that it was too early to assume the swine flu outbreak was mild because no one in the UK had died, and that there may be a resurgence of the virus in autumn and winter.

It was confirmed on 28 May that a man in Scotland is critically ill with swine flu. He has other health problems. There are now four people now critically ill and in intensive care, all from Scotland.

Outbreak Timeline

2009	*UK Swine Flu Outbreak Milestone*
27 Apr.	First two UK H1N1 cases confirmed in Scotland after a flight from Mexico.
29 Apr.	Paignton Community and Sports College closes for about a week in first school closure.
1 May	First two UK person to person transmissions confirmed.
2 May	Further schools are temporarily closed from this date.
7 May	HPA issues advice on exclusion from schools and workplaces.
8 May	HPA issues "advice on actions to be taken in a school in the event of a probable or confirmed case of "swine flu" being

	identified in a school pupil", in which closure for 7 days is advised when appropriate.
	The virus from European samples isolated and its full genetic fingerprint determined by UK researchers, following similar work in the US on the virus in the American continent.
11 May	First two schools closed reopen.
17 May	One hundredth confirmed case.
19 May	More than half of the UK cases are in London, and more than half are contracted in the UK.
22 May	HPA staff no longer routinely meet flights from Mexico. Contact tracing of passengers deemed to be at risk of swine flu carried out on the basis of risk, as for other communicable diseases.
26 May	The largest single outbreak so far, with 50 confirmed cases identified at a Birmingham primary school (later increased to 74).
31 May	The first case confirmed in Wales.
6 June	More than 500 confirmed cases in the UK.

Reported Cases

Detailed Reports: On April 25, 2009, a member of British Airways cabin crew was taken to Northwick Park Hospital in Harrow and quarantined after falling ill with flu-like symptoms on a flight from Mexico City though he was later found not to have swine flu.

On 26 April, two people were admitted to Monklands Hospital in Airdrie, North Lanarkshire, with mild flu-like symptoms after returning from Mexico. The next day, the Cabinet Secretary for Health and Wellbeing, Nicola Sturgeon, confirmed that these were cases of the swine influenza A (H1N1) virus. The two people involved were later named as Iain and Dawn Askham, a newly-married couple who had been on their honeymoon in the resort of Cancun in the Mexican Caribbean. Authorities in both Scotland and England stated that there were no plans to trace the fellow airline passengers who may have travelled alongside the couple, since the authorities do not classify them as "close contacts".

These cases along with one in Spain are the first confirmed cases in Europe.

At noon on 29 April the government officially made public three more confirmed cases in the UK, including the first cases in England. These were two adults (one in Redditch, and one in London), and a 12-year-old girl in Torbay, Devon. All three new cases had recently arrived back from Mexico. The girl's school, Paignton Community and Sports College, closed for seven days as a result of her diagnosis.

On 30 April, Newcastle University advised their students and staff of a confirmed case in a household where a non-student shares a property with two students, antiviral drugs were administered and the university stayed open. The total number of new confirmed cases for 30 April was three, one on Newcastle and two more in London.

The first UK person-to-person transmission was confirmed on 1 May. The victim, from Falkirk, was infected after contact with the first Britons to develop the flu. The same day it was confirmed that a 12-year-old girl from Downend in South Gloucestershire had been diagnosed with swine flu. She was on the same flight as the Scottish couple who tested positive earlier in the week. A 42-year-old man, in South Gloucestershire, is the second "onward transmission" case in the United Kingdom; officials said the two Gloucestershire cases were not connected. The man, who lives in Chipping Sodbury, was believed to have caught the virus from someone who had visited Mexico or United States.

On 2 May the Department of Health confirmed that an adult in the North West and a child in the South East had contracted the virus. The total number of UK confirmed cases stood at 15.

On 3 May, Scottish health authorities reported a case in Ayrshire, where a man reportedly caught the virus in the US state of Texas.

On 4 May nine new cases were confirmed. Two cases are adults, from London and the West Midlands. Both of these cases had recently returned from Mexico. Two cases are siblings of school age in London, who are close contacts of a previously confirmed case in a returned traveller to the US. Five further cases are of school age from London. These five all attend one school.

On 5 May one new case was confirmed in South East England, a traveller returning from Mexico.

Since then and as of 23 May there have been a few new cases (only once more than 10) confirmed every day, a few hundreds under investigation, and no deaths. Most UK cases are in London. A large proportion of cases are from person-to-person infection within the UK, but the HPA daily updates include a significant minority of travellers infected elsewhere.

As of 26 May, The majority of cases were in school children and young adults and the number of people who contracted the disease in-country increased to 125, Which is the highest in Europe and triple the second highest, Spain, Which has 42 people who have contracted the disease in-country.

On 28 May, sixty four people connected with a primary school in Birmingham have being diagnosed with Swine Flu. To this date, it was the biggest single outbreak of Swine Flu in the United Kingdom.

On 2 June the Health Department announced two new critical patients in Renfrewshire, Scotland. One is wholly due to swine flu.

On 3 of June the number of cases of swine flu risen to 64 to 88 in a day, 4 are now critically ill, in Scotland

On 8 June the HPA issued a report stating that the majority of cases are in school age children and young adults, which has not been the case in most pandemics with the notable exception of 1918.

Public Information Campaign

The Department of Health announced on 29 April 2009 that they intended to send an information leaflet on swine flu to every household in the UK. On 5 May they started to deliver leaflets to all households in the UK. On 29 April, Alan Johnson announced that television and radio advice would also be broadcast starting on 30 April. On 30 April 2009, a swine flu information line was launched with advice on setting up "flu friends".

The Department of Health Pandemic Plan (revised November 2007) states "UK health departments (directorate in Scotland) will run a national door drop and advertising campaign in Phase 5, alerting the public to the heightened risk, emphasising the need for personal preparation and socially responsible behaviour. A public information film will demonstrate how to slow the spread of the virus, and the National Flu Line service will be available. Information materials will also be available through primary care, pharmacies and on the Department of Health website." The National Flu Line service is due to be launched in late-2009.

There are government websites with general information and the latest updates on human swine flu in the UK, Northern Ireland, Scotland, and Wales.

The HPA website includes frequently updated advice for the public, advice on exclusion from schools and workplaces (and a document specifically for schools), and information for health professionals.

Controlling Measures

As of 11 May 2009 UK epidemiologists at Imperial College London consider that H1N1 swine flu is spreading fast enough to justify the preparations for a pandemic. It is showing "sustained human-to-human transmission", thereby justifying the WHO's pandemic phase 5 rating. It is estimated that on average each person who contracts flu passes it on to between 1.4 and 1.6 other people, no worse than the three influenza pandemics of the twentieth century. Early analysis suggests that the spread is likely to be similar to the earlier pandemics. Up to the date of the study, clinical severity is similar to 1957 and less than 1918. However, the clinical severity of the outbreak and how the virus will evolve cannot yet be predicted.

Travel to and from Affected Areas

On 27 April, the Foreign and Commonwealth Office advised against all but essential travel to Mexico and stated that British citizens in Mexico... "may wish to consider whether they should remain in Mexico at this time". On 28 April the Mexican Tourist Board estimated that there were "a few thousand" British tourists in Mexico.

British Airways is continuing to fly to Mexico City four times per week. It is offering passengers the option of cancelling their flights, or rebooking to another destination with no cancellation fees.

Holiday companies Thomas Cook and Airtours said that between them they had about "3,000 holidaymakers in Mexico" as of 28 April 2009. The first British tourists being brought back early from Mexico on 28 April 2009 told reporters that they had received little or no information about health precautions, either from the Mexican authorities, hotels, or from local tour guides.

A leaflet is being distributed at all ports of entry into the UK providing passengers arriving in the UK with information on swine flu.

Until 21 May HPA staff met travellers arriving from Mexico. This was discontinued on 22 May, but advice remained that travellers from affected areas who become unwell within seven days of arrival, and contacts with symptoms of a confirmed or probable case, should stay at home and contact their GP or NHS Direct. Contact tracing of passengers deemed to be at risk of swine flu will be carried out on the basis of risk, as for other communicable diseases.

Preparations: Information, advice, and guidance both general and for specific cases (schools, workplaces) is being made available and updated by the HPA.

On 27 April, UK health secretary Alan Johnson stated that Britain has a stockpile of 33 million courses of antiviral drugs effective against this strain, enough for one course for around half of the UK's population. On 30 April, Alan Johnson stated that the government was obtaining extra antiviral drugs that would protect 50 million people, amounting to more than three-quarters of the UK population.

There is a pandemic plan covering topics from distributing the drugs and setting up helplines to closing schools and banning public events which was tested in a large exercise in 2007. There is also a specific response plan for London.

It should be noted that oseltamivir (Tamiflu) and zanamivir (Relenza), the two antivirals known to be effective, must be taken within 48 hours of onset of symptoms or earlier to be effective; the positive effects are greatest if treatment is started within six hours. To be effective stockpiled supplies must be made available to patients within this timescale, regardless of weekends and holidays.

On 5 May 2009 plans were announced for pupils unable to sit examinations at schools affected by flu to be assessed in other ways to ensure that children are not disadvantaged.

Testing Suspected Cases

Genetic Analysis: Samples from suspected cases have been analysed by the National Institute for Medical Research in London, which is also examining samples of the US strain of the disease.

By 8 May 2009 the US Centres for Disease Control and Prevention had made genetic information on the swine flu virus available, and the virus from European samples had been isolated and its full genetic fingerprint determined by UK researchers. The genetics and effects of the virus in general are discussed in the article on the 2009 swine flu outbreak.

Diagnosis: The fastest way for laboratory confirmation of swine flu is by the PCR method, described as a real-time method. According to the WHO there are four laboratories in the UK able to perform PCR to diagnose influenza A (H1N1) virus infection in humans: Regional Virus Laboratory, Royal Victoria Hospital, Belfast, NI; Regional Virus Laboratory, Gartnavel General Hospital, Glasgow, Scotland; Health Protection Agency, Centre for Infections, Enteric, Respiratory, and Neurological Virus Laboratory, London; WHO Collaborating Centre for Reference and Research on Influenza, National Institute for Medical Research, London.

Another laboratory confirmation is a fourfold increase in virus-specific antibodies 10 to 14 days later.

Hygiene Recommendations

The Health Protection Agency in guidance included in its regular updates recommends infection control practices and good hygiene to help reduce transmission of all viruses, including swine flu. These include:

- Covering nose and mouth when coughing or sneezing, and using a tissue when possible.
- Disposing of dirty tissues promptly and carefully.
- Maintaining good basic hygiene, for example washing hands frequently with soap and water to reduce the spread of the virus from your hands to face or to other people.
- Cleaning hard surfaces, such as door handles, frequently using a normal cleaning product.
- Making sure children follow this advice.
- Anyone with swine flu or being investigated as a possible case will be given antivirals and asked to stay at home and limit their contact with other people.
- Where antivirals are prescribed the course of treatment must be followed and completed, although it may sometimes cause nausea.

Professor Steve Field, chairman of the Royal College of General Practitioners, said on 28 April that people in the UK were *"perfectly safe at the moment"*, and did not need to start wearing facemasks or stop eating pork.

Possible Use of Facemasks

Home Secretary (formerly Health Secretary) Alan Johnson told MPs on 27 April that "Although we are aware that facemasks are being given out to the public in Mexico, the available scientific evidence does not support the general wearing of facemasks by those who are not ill, whilst going about their normal activities."

Professor Steve Field, chairman of the Royal College of General Practitioners, said people in the UK were "perfectly safe at the moment", and did not need to start wearing facemasks or stop eating pork.

The Head of Pandemic Planning at the Royal College of General Practitioners, Dr. Maureen Baker, stated on 27 April that "Masks become ineffective when they become damp or after a few hours. There has been a lot of debate on the use of facemasks and some authorities say that, in the community, the most effective use is to give to patients who may have symptoms when they present in the surgery — that should help reduce the infectivity of that patient to surgery staff and other patients. I expect the Department of Health will issue guidance on use of facemasks if we move into a pandemic phase." Masks may not protect the wearer from inhalation of the virus, but might protect other people from picking up the virus from the wearer.

Professor John Oxford, a virologist at leading London hospital, The Barts and the London, said: "Really, there is very little evidence that masks actually offer much protection against flu.

It is reported that the UK government is urgently seeking to acquire more facemasks.

North America

In Canada, as of May 26, there has been 2 deaths and a further 921 confirmed cases of swine flu, most of which was contracted in-country, have been confirmed in the country; 68 in Nova Scotia, 114 in British Columbia, 86 in Alberta, 284 in

Ontario, 106 in Quebec, 2 in New Brunswick, 6 in Manitoba, 3 in Prince Edward Island, 49 in Saskatchewan, and 1 in Yukon Territory. The country's first four cases, in Nova Scotian students who had travelled to Mexico, were confirmed on April 26. On April 30, the first case of swine flu affecting someone who had not travelled to Mexico was confirmed in Nova Scotia. On May 8, the first confirmed death from the H1N1 virus was reported in Alberta.

Dr. Jose Angel Cordova Villalobos, Mexico's Secretariat of Health, stated that since March 2009, there have been over 1,995 suspected cases and 149 deaths, with 20 confirmed to be linked to a new swine influenza strain of Influenza A virus subtype H1N1. "'As many as 23,000 Mexicans were likely infected with the swine flu virus,' Neil Ferguson of Imperial College London and colleagues reported in the journal Science."

Soldiers mobilised by the government have handed out six million surgical masks to citizens in and around Mexico City. On April 24, 2009, schools (from pre-school to university level) as well as libraries, museums, concerts and any public gathering place, were shut down by the government in Mexico City and the neighbouring State of Mexico to prevent the disease from spreading further; the schools in Mexico City, the State of Mexico, and the state of San Luis Potosi will remain closed until at least May 5. Marcelo Ebrard, Mexico City's mayor, has also asked all night-life operators to shut down their places of business for ten days to prevent further infections.

On April 25, President Felipe Calderon declared an emergency which granted him the power to suspend public events and order quarantines. On April 26, the World Bank announced US$ 25 million in immediate aid loans to Mexico, an additional US$ 180 million for long-term assistance to address the outbreak, and advice on how other nations have responded to similar crises. On April 27, the Secretariat of Public Education announced that all schools in Mexico will remain closed at least until May 6. On April 28, the Mexico City government closed all restaurants and cinemas. The National History and

Anthropology Institute also closed all its archaeological sites and museums, including the most famous Mayan and Aztec ruins, until further notice.

In the United States, initial reports of atypical flu in two individuals in southern California led to the discovery of the novel swine flu virus by the CDC in mid-April. More than a hundred cases were confirmed in the next two weeks, spread through a dozen states.

Outside of California and Texas, initial cases were all tied to recent travel to Mexico or close contact with those who had recently visited Mexico. St. Francis Preparatory School, a private school in New York, was the centre of a large cluster of cases after a Spring Break trip by several students, and perforce one of the first US schools to be closed as a public health measure during the early outbreak. Most of the cases in California and Texas are not linked and may reflect localised outbreaks of this virus in those areas.

The disease was not as virulent outside of Mexico as within Mexico, for reasons not fully understood. The US declared a state of Public Health Emergency but this was said to be standard procedure in cases as divergent as the recent inauguration and flooding. On April 29, the US suffered its first confirmed death of swine flu, and on May 5 the first US citizen died from swine flu. As of June 6, there were 17 confirmed deaths from swine flu in the US. As of mid-May 2009 many states had abandoned testing for likely influenza cases unless serious illness and/or hospitalisation were present.

Because reported numbers represent only confirmed cases, they are a "very great understatement" of the total number of cases of infection, according to the CDC. The real number of swine flu cases in the United States could be "upwards of 100,000," a top public health official estimated on Friday — far higher than the official count of 7,415 cases confirmed by laboratories. The United States now has more than 12000 confirmed cases and more than 30 deaths due to swine flu.

Caribbean

In Aruba, all passengers arriving by airplane or cruise ship were required to fill out a health questionnaire beginning on April 27, 2009. Hotels and resorts are required to report to authorities if any tourists are showing flu-like symptoms. The government of Aruba also ordered antiviral medication and other supplies from the Netherlands and the United States. No swine flu cases have been reported. In Barbados, two samples were sent to Trinidad and Tobago to be tested for the virus.

Cuba suspended flights to and from Mexico for 48 hours. The first case of swine flu in Cuba was confirmed in mid-May.

The first two cases in the Dominican Republic were confirmed on May 27. On June 5, a 17-year-old pregnant girl infected with the AH1N1 virus died. 66 cases were confirmed to this date.

As of 31 May 2009, there has been seven confirmed cases of swine flu in Jamaica. Health Minister Ruddy Spencer told Parliament that the country has been placed on high alert. There has been heightened surveillance at health care facilities and port entry's.

One female has been confirmed as having contracted the H1N1 influenza.

In the Bahamas, ten students and teachers who arrived from Mexico in the last week of April are in quarantine.

Central America

In Belize, there were two suspected cases of swine flu under investigation. As a result, all major public events were cancelled.

The first two cases of swine flu in Costa Rica, both of whom had travelled to Mexico, were confirmed on April 28. Since April 29 the Ministry of Health recommended to avoid travel to Mexico, Canada, and the US. A 53 year-old man became the first confirmed death from the disease in the country, as reported on May 9. By June 5 the Costa Rican Ministry of

Health had 83 confirmed cases of influenza A (H1N1) leading to one fatality, two probable cases pending confirmation, 107 suspected cases, and 1,506 already discarded.

Guatemala is checking all travellers arriving from Mexico for signs of flu and stopping anyone with symptoms of the virus at border crossings. On May 5, in a meeting with Health Minister and the Vice President, it was announced that an 11-year-old girl was infected with the AH1N1 virus.

Honduras reported its first confirmed case of swine flu (H1N1) on 27 May, 2009. By June 7 the country had reported 67 cases of H1N1 Influenza, most of the cases on the city of San Pedro Sula and the Atlantic Coastline. There are few cases on other cities and areas. All airports and commercial sites as well as public events are monitored.

As on June 4, *179 confirmed cases* had been reported by Panamanian health authorities. Of these, 91 were male and 88 were female. Schools with positive cases are being disinfected. Thermal cameras had been deployed in Tocument Int'l Airpot to identify sickness in arriving passengers.

Swine Flu Outbreak in Oceania 2009

Australia: As of June 5, 2009, Australia has more than 1,000 confirmed cases, at least two of which were contracted in country. The alert level has been lifted from "delay" to "contain", giving authorities in all states the option to close schools if students are at risk.

Australia has a stockpile of 8.7 million doses of Tamiflu and Relenza. Airlines have been required to report passengers from the Americas with influenza symptoms, and nurses have been deployed at international airports.

On May 9, the first confirmed case in Australia was reported.

On May 20, four additional cases were reported, one in New South Wales and three in Victoria.

On May 21, an additional case was reported in Victoria. Victorian health authorities close Clifton Hill Primary School for two days (initially) after three brothers return to the school from a trip to Disneyland and are confirmed to have H1N1

On May 22, cases were reported in South Australian and Victoria, including the first reported cases where the virus was contracted in Australia.

On May 25, the first confirmed case in Western Australia was reported.

On May 26, 3 additional cases were reported in Sydney. The newly confirmed cases involved two children who arrived in Sydney on the cruise ship named Pacific Dawn and another child who had recently returned from a trip to the United States. NSW Health issued a directive to the 2000 passengers who arrived in Sydney on the Pacific Dawn requiring that they stay at home for 7 days.

Fiji: Fiji on Wednesday moved to high alert against the swine flu virus, with the authorities admitting the Pacific island nation was not immune to the rapidly spreading global threat.

On Thursday April 30, 2009, a traveller suspected of being infected by the swine flu virus is under close surveillance at Lautoka Hospital, said the Health Ministry. Hours later, the Health Ministry said there are two suspected cases.

French Polynesia: French Polynesia has reported no cases of swine flu so far. Officials installed a thermal imaging camera on April 27, 2009, at Faa'a International Airport in Tahiti to screen all arriving international passengers. French Polynesia has 48,000 Tamiflu antiviral treatments available in case of an outbreak, and more can be flown into Tahiti within twenty-four hours.

New Caledonia: On June 2, 2009 the authorities in New Caledonia refused to allow the cruise-ship from Australia, the *Dawn Princess* to dock because five patients on board had flu-like symptoms.

New Zealand: The impact in New Zealand has been almost negligible with no fatalities reported in this country. There is no evidence of community transmission in New Zealand. All of the cases are people who have recently returned from travelling to affected areas, or are close contacts of known cases.

On Saturday April the 25th 2009 ten students from Rangitoto College, a secondary school in North Shore City, Auckland, exhibited influenza symptoms on returning from a three week language trip to Mexico. All 22 students and three accompanying teachers from the trip and those in close contact with them were placed in voluntary home isolation and treated with oseltamivir. The ten students tested positive for an influenza A virus, with three of them later testing positive for swine flu. The symptoms were reportedly mild and all affected individuals have since recovered.

New Zealand has had a well developed Influenza Pandemic action plan since 2006. Following this plan New Zealand immediately upgraded its influenza pandemic alert status to code yellow. The national stockpile of 1.4 million doses of oseltamivir was released to regional health authorities. The initial response as specified in the Pandemic Action Plan is a policy of border control and cluster control via voluntary quarantine and treatment of contacts with oseltamivir. As of May 24, this policy appears to have been successful in preventing the Mexican Flu from spreading within New Zealand.

As of May 30, New Zealand has had 9 laboratory confirmed cases and 10 probable cases. All have since recovered. There has been no substantive change to these figures since May 15. New Zealand continues to identify isolate and treat suspected cases. There are currently 30 suspected cases and 23 people are in isolation being treated with Tamiflu. Confirmed cases have tested positive for the Mexican swine flu strain of influenza type A. Probable cases have tested positive for influenza type A after possible recent exposure to the Mexican strain. Suspected cases have flu symptoms after possible recent exposure to the Mexican strain. On June 6 a one-year-old boy from Manukau City was diagnosed with swine flu and several other people who had been exposed to him had gone into isolation.

On June 8, the Ministry of Health confirmed three further cases of novel Influenza A(H1N1); bringing the national total to 17. One of the new cases is the son of a Canterbury man who recently flew into New Zealand on Air NZ flight NZ5. The other two new cases came from international flights from Los Angeles (NZ5) and Melbourne (NZ124). These people have been isolated and are being treated with Tamiflu. Health officials are in the process of contacted those who may have had contact with those confirmed of having Influenza A(H1N1).

New Zealand had about 48,000 influenza cases in the 2008 flu season – 42 per cent of which were type A – and approximately 100 deaths a year directly attributed to influenza viruses.

Palau: Palau has issued a health alert for swine flu.

Health Minister Dr. Stevenson Kuartei told reporters that although there is no reported case in Palau, a Task Force has been convened to increase screening of passengers entering the country.

Solomon Islands: A multi-sectoral task force has been activated by the Solomon Islands Ministry of Health to deal with the swine influenza virus.

Permanent Secretary of the Ministry of Health and Medical Service Lester Ross said a task force is managing the Solomon Island Ministry of health's response to recent threat of swine flu epidemic.

Tokelau: Most supplies and food shipments to Tokelau are sent by ferry from the neighbouring country of Samoa. The Samoa Health Ministry had cancelled all travel to Tokelau until further notice as a precaution against the introduction of swine flu to the Tokelauan population. The Operations Manager for the Tokelau Office in Apia, Samoa, Makalio Ioane, confirmed that some ferry travel would still be allowed to Tokelau, but the ship's crew would not be allowed to leave the boat or dock in Tokelau. The boat will be off loaded without any physical contact with the Tokelauan population. No cases of swine flu have been reported on either Tokelau or Samoa, so the cessation of travel to Tokelau is considered a precaution.

Tonga: Tonga has set up an Emergency Taskforce and is performing screen checks at its International Airport for passengers experiencing influenza symptoms, most importantly from flights originating from Los Angeles.

Nauru: One suspected case of swine flu has been identified in Nauru. Travellers entering Nauru are now screened for influenza symptoms, most importantly from flights originating from North America.

Vanuatu: Travellers entering the country via Santo-Pekoa International Airport and Bauerfield International Airport are now being screened using body heat detection before being allowed to exit the airport's gates.

On June 5, one 6-week-old infant has been confirmed to have died from swine flu in Vanuatu.

Swine Flu Outbreak in South America 2009

On April 2009, an outbreak of a new strain of influenza hit Mexico and the United States. The new strain was identified as a combination of several different strains of Influenzavirus A, subtype H1N1, including separate strains of this subtype circulating in humans and in pigs.

On 3 May 2009, the first case of the flu was confirmed in the continent in a Colombian man who recently travelled from Mexico since then it has extended to the entire region, excluding The Guianas, for a total of 1330 cases including two deaths. By far, the most affected country had been Chile with 890 cases and 2 deaths.

The World Health Organisation warned about the arrival of the southern winter in the southern hemisphere, where there are seasonal peaks of flu, that could increase the number of infections

Argentina: According to an Epidemic Alert order issued by the Ministry of Health, Airlines have been required to report passengers with influenza symptoms arriving from Mexico and United States. Passengers from these countries must fill out a form to be located should they experience any symptoms. In addition, the government has also stepped up safety checks, and thermal scanners are being used on airports to detect passengers with fever and other influenza symptoms. As of April 28, the Government has suspended all flights originated from Mexico until May 15 as a precautionary measure.

On May 7, Health Authorities confirmed the first case, a tourist that had recently returned from Mexico. 55 other suspected cases continue to be studied under isolation.

On May 22, Health Authorities confirmed the second case, a woman who had arrived from the United States about 20 days ago.

At May 23, there were 221 possible cases, two have been confirmed, 173 were negative for influenza A (H1N1) and 46 cases are under study.

On May 24, three more cases were confirmed.

On May 25, 14 more cases were confirmed, increasing the number of cases to 19.

On May 27, 18 more cases were confirmed, increasing the number of cases to 37.

On May 28, 33 more cases were confirmed, increasing the number of cases to 70.

On May 29, 10 more cases were confirmed, increasing the number of cases to 80.

On May 30, 20 more cases were confirmed, bringing the total cases to 100. There were suspected 371 cases being studied.

On May 31, 15 more cases were confirmed, bringing the number of cases to 115.

On June 1, 16 more cases were confirmed, increasing the number of cases to 131.

Brazil: Two people who had arrived in Brazil from Mexico with symptoms of an undefined illness were hospitalised in

Sao Paulo on April 25. It was initially suspected that they were suffering from the swine flu virus. The Brazilian Ministry of Health later issued a press release stating that while the exact cause of the two patients illnesses remained unknown, they *"did not meet the definition of suspected cases of swine influenza because they did not have signs and symptoms consistent with the disease: fever over 39 °C, accompanied by coughing and/or a headache, muscle and joint pain."*

The press release also stated that airports would monitor travellers arriving from affected areas, under the direction of the National Sanitary Surveillance Agency (ANVISA). Air crews were trained on signs and symptoms of swine influenza so that passengers displaying symptoms would receive guidance from ANVISA upon arrival.

On May 30, the Minister said that the country has 20 confirmed cases, 8 in Sao Paulo, 5 in Rio de Janeiro, 4 in Santa Catarina, 1 in Minas Gerais, 1 in Rio Grande do Sul and 1 in Tocantins. Three of the 5 cases in Rio are of transmission inside the country and two of the four in Santa Catarina are two.

On June 2, 3 more cases were confirmed, one in Sao Paulo and two in Rio de Janeiro, increasing the number of cases to 23.

On June 4, the number of confirmed cases increase to 28 with another 3 in Sao Paulo and 2 in Mato Grosso do Sul.

Chile: On April 27, the Assistant Secretary of Health Jeanette Vega, confirmed that there are eight suspected cases of swine influenza in the country, which are being examined at the Hospital del Torax in Santiago. Five other cases have been dismissed by the authorities.

On April 28 the Health Ministry announced 26 cases under investigation: 16 in Santiago; 2 in Atacama; 2 in Valparaiso; 4 in O'Higgins Region; 1 in Biobio and 1 in Araucania. 16 other cases have been dismissed.

On May 1, the Health Ministry announced that it continued to investigate 4 suspected cases: 2 in Santiago, 1 in Valparaiso and 1 in Araucania. To date, 80 suspected cases have been examined by the Health Ministry; 76 of those have been dismissed. Another suspected case was identified on May 2, bringing the number of cases under investigation to 5.

On May 10, the Health Ministry announced that 116 cases have been dismissed, and there are no cases pending test results.

On May 17, the Chilean Health Minister confirmed, the first case of A(H1N1) flu in Chile, the same day two more cases were confirmed

On May 29, the Chilean Health ministry confirmed the number of cases of A-H1N1 had risen to 224., the same day two more cases were confirmed.

On June 3 Chile suffered its first confirmed death of swine flu. A 37-year-old man from Puerto Montt.

Colombia: The Minister of Social Protection, Diego Palacio Betancourt, announced on April 26, 2009, that 12 suspect cases had been detected, 9 in Bogota and 3 on the Caribbean coast. Samples of the virus have been sent to the USA for comparisons and analysis. Results of the testing were expected within few days. On April 27, the Government declared a "national disaster" state in order to face the emergency, which allowed health authorities to have a special budget to do so. As of April 28, most of the suspect cases were excluded, with only four remaining: three Mexican teachers in Bogotá, and one person in Cartagena. Another 38 suspect cases were under observation. On April 29, the suspect cases raised to 49, with 10 of them "highly" suspect. The government purchased 400,000 oseltamivir (Tamiflu) doses, which will be distributed through the Social Protection ministry to the affected if there are confirmed cases.

On May 3, 2009, Minister Palacio confirmed the first case of A(H1N1) in Colombia, in a 42-year-old person from Zipaquirá, who recently travelled to Mexico. According to Palacio, only one out of 18 tests sent to Atlanta was positive. The patient was isolated and put under medical treatment. On the same day, Palacio stated there were 108 suspect cases in the country.

Ecuador: Health officials are carrying out checks on people with flu symptoms entering the country from sea or air. On April 29, Ecuador closed its borders to Mexican citizens and foreigners of other nationalities arriving from Mexico for a period of 30 days. On May 15, Health officials confirmed the first case of AH1N1 flu in Ecuador . On May 20, the Health Department confirmed 7 more new cases of AH1N1, raising the total number of infected people to 8, the number has now risen to 41.

Paraguay: Paraguay is the country with the least number of cases in the continent and the Minister of Health stated that the situation is under control. As of June 1, the number of confirmed cases is still at 5.

Peru: The Governor of Callao, Alex Kouri, ordered that all passengers from any infected country, mainly Mexico, Canada and USA, must be checked before their arrival on Peruvian territory. Also, the Peruvian government must be warned of any case or symptom of fever. This step is in order to prevent any infections, since the main port and airport of Peru are located in Callao. Also, the government has prepared a special area at the Hospital "Daniel Alcides Carrion" to treat cases of this disease.

The first suspicious case has been detected in the morning of April 27, 2009. It was a Peruvian woman who returned from Mexico.

In Peru 5 people were considered suspects with the virus, but as of April 28 have been confirmed to be healthy and not carrying the H1N1 virus. The government has stated that the country is clean, but efforts are being made to examine slaughterhouses and they are screening incoming passengers from problem areas.

On April 29, Peru's Health Minister Oscar Ugarte confirmed one case of swine flu. On April 30, he said the case is not entirely confirmed. Having recently visited Mexico, the patient was flying in a Copa Airlines airplane from Panama to Buenos Aires on April 28, but the flight was diverted to Lima due to her illness.

The crew only notified of the suspicion of swine flu only after the passenger had checked in the airport. Three more suspected cases were being investigated. Ugarte also announced the suspension of all commercial flights from Mexico to Peru. On May 14, Ugarte totally confirmed a case of swine flu from a peruvian woman who returned from New York, plus another suspected case in Trujillo from another woman in the same flight. On May 17, the second case was confirmed, an American born man residing in Arequipa. He had returned from the US on May 12, not showing any symptoms until two days later.

On May 18 a new case was confirmed, a scholar returning from a trip to Dominican Republic, that studied in the Altair school. Classes for her class in that school had being suspended until May 25. 19 May, another case of a scholar from the same trip to Dominican Republic. Student had contact with 3rd victim and both studied in the same school.

Uruguay: Uruguay confirmed its first two cases on May 27 in a 27-year-old man and a 15 year woman who recently arrived from Argentina.

As of June 5 a total of 21 people have been infected with the virus.

Venezuela: Controls have been raised at airports to prevent contagion from spreading. Travellers from the United States and Mexico with flu symptoms are being isolated until they are given the all clear. Pig farms in the country are being "closely inspected" and stockpiles of medicines built up.

On May 28 the Health Minister, Jesus Mantilla, confirmed the first case of the A/H1N1 flu in a Venezuelan citizen who arrived in a flight from Panama four days ago. He was isolated to the place he is receiving treatment and his condition is stable. . The following day, a second case was confirmed from another person who also arrived from the same flight. On June 1 another case was tested positive and was also linked to the previous two cases. On June 3 a fourth case was confirmed from a male citizen who arrived from Brazil. The Minister of Health confirmed that all the patients are stable and there is no need to alarm the population.

On June 8, the number of confirmed cases increased to 12 also from citizens who arrived from Panama, France and the USA. Later that day a 13th case was confirmed, this time an 9-year-old boy who recently came from Colombia.

12

Influenza Research

Influenza research involves investigating molecular virology, pathogeneses, host immune responses, genomics, and epidemiology regarding influenza. The main goal of research is to develop influenza countermeasures such as vaccines, therapies and diagnostic tools.

The potential H5N1 pandemic has motivated a huge increase in flu research. At least 12 companies and 17 governments are developing pre-pandemic influenza vaccines in 28 different clinical trials that, if successful, could turn a deadly pandemic infection into a non-deadly pandemic infection. A vaccine that could prevent any illness at all from the not-yet-existing pandemic influenza strain will take at least three months from the virus's emergence until full-scale vaccine production could begin; with vaccine production hoped to increase until one billion doses are produced by one year after the virus is first identified.

Improved influenza countermeasures require basic research on how viruses enter cells, replicate, mutate, evolve into new strains and induce an immune response. Solutions to limitations in current vaccine methods are being researched.

The Influenza Genome Sequencing Project is creating a library of influenza sequences that will help us understand what makes one strain more lethal than another, what genetic determinants most affect immunogenicity, and how the virus evolves over time.

Areas of Current Flu Research

Before 2004, all previous highly pathogenic avian flu virus strains circulated only among domesticated poultry and by culling all of them in the area, the strains were made extinct. Previous HPAI strains only existed in domesticated birds. A wild bird's LPAI would mutate in a domestic flock into an HPAI strain, all domestic birds in the area would be killed, and the HPAI strain would no longer have any hosts and thus would no longer exist.

This current HPAI H5N1 strain has turned out to be different. In October 2004 researchers discovered H5N1 is far more dangerous than previously believed because waterfowl, especially ducks, were directly spreading the highly pathogenic strain of H5N1. From this point on, avian flu experts increasingly referred to containment as a strategy that can delay but not prevent a future avian flu pandemic.

Nonetheless, there is still hope it will mutate into some low pathogenic strain over time and no longer exist in its current high pathogenic set of strains. But as time as gone on, the hope has come to look less and less likely. The result is that billions of dollars every year are going to be needed in expenditures that would not be required if it did go away. Poultry farming is especially hard hit. How to best spend pandemic mitigation funds and poultry farming protection funds is a question that to be answered requires billions in flu research and new flu vaccine manufacturing factories.

Since it is not going away as was hoped, more data is needed to figure out how best to cope. So governments are funding a variety of studies from cell culture of flu viruses to H5N1 vaccination effectiveness to adjuvants to wild bird migration patterns to wild bird avian flu subtype distribution to poultry flu vaccination, etc. The information being gathered is increasing the world's ability to keep H5N1 contained, limiting its speed and extent of mutation, and buying time for new flu vaccine manufacturing methods and factories to come on line so that when the next flu pandemic happens the death toll can be minimised.

Current Major Flu Research Contracts

The US federal government on May 4, 2006 awarded five-year contracts for "more than $1 billion to five drug manufacturers developing technology for speedier mass production of vaccines in the event of a pandemic" from the $3.8 billion pandemic preparedness bill passed in 2005. "The federal government says its goal is to be able to distribute a vaccine to every American within six months of a pandemic. Currently, flu vaccines are produced in specialised chicken eggs, but that technique does not allow for speedy mass vaccinations." The companies receiving the contracts were:

- GlaxoSmithKline $274.8 million;
- MedImmune Inc. $169.5 million;
- Novartis Vaccines and Diagnostics $220.5 million;
- DynPort Vaccine Company, LLC $41 million;
- Solvay Pharmaceuticals $298.6 million.

The US government has purchased from Sanofi Pasteur and Chiron Corporation several million doses of vaccine meant to be use in case of an influenza pandemic from H5N1 and is conducting clinical trials on them. ABC News reported on April 1, 2006 that "Beginning in late-1997, the human trials have tested 30 different vaccines, all pegged to the H5N1 virus."

To address the H9N2 threat, NIAID contracted with Chiron Corporation to produce investigational batches of an inactivated vaccine, which will be evaluated clinically by NIAID early next year. For H5N1, Aventis-Pasteur and Chiron are both producing investigational lots of inactivated H5N1 vaccine preparations; additionally, DHHS has contracted with Aventis to produce up to 2 million doses to be stockpiled for emergency use, if needed, to vaccinate health workers, researchers, and, if indicated, the public in affected areas. Development and evaluation of a combination antiviral regimen against these potential pandemic influenza strains are also now under way.

Vaccines

A vaccine probably would not be available in the initial stages of population infection . Once a potential virus is identified, it normally takes at least several months before a vaccine becomes widely available, as it must be developed, tested and authorised. The capability to produce vaccines varies widely from country to country; in fact, only 15 countries are listed as "Influenza vaccine manufacturers" according to the World Health Organisation .

It is estimated that, in a best scenario situation, 750 million doses could be produced each year, whereas it is likely that each individual would need two doses of the vaccine in order to become immuno-competent. Distribution to and inside countries would probably be problematic . Several countries, however, have well-developed plans for producing large quantities of vaccine. For example, Canadian health authorities say that they are developing the capacity to produce 32 million doses within four months, enough vaccine to inoculate every person in the country.

There are two serious technical problems associated with the development of a vaccine against H5N1. The first problem is this: seasonal influenza vaccines require a single injection of 15 mg haemagglutinin in order to give protection; H5 seems to evoke only a weak immune response and a large multicentre trial found that two injections of 90 μg H5 given 28 days apart provided protection in only 54 per cent of people (Treanor 2006). Even if it is considered that 54 per cent is an acceptable level of protection, the world is currently capable of producing only 900 million doses at a strength of 15 mg (assuming that all production were immediately converted to manufacturing H5 vaccine); if two injections of 90 mg are needed then this capacity drops to only 70 million (Poland 2006). Trials using adjuvants such as alum or MF59 to try and lower the dose of vaccine are urgently needed. The second problem is this: there are two circulating clades of virus, clade 1 is the virus originally isolated in Vietnam, clade 2 is the virus isolated in Indonesia. Current vaccine research is focused on clade 1 viruses, but the clade 2 virus is antigenically distinct and a clade 1 vaccine will probably not protect against a pandemic caused by clade 2 virus.

Live Attenuated Influenza Vaccine

In June 2007, the National Institutes of Health (NIH) began enrolling participants in a Phase 1 H5N1 study of an intranasal influenza vaccine candidate based on Flumist, MedImmune's live, attenuated vaccine technology.

Reverse Genetics

A technique called reverse genetics allows scientists to manipulate the genomes of influenza viruses and to transfer genes between viral strains. The technique allows the rapid generation of seed viruses for vaccine candidates that exactly match the anticipated epidemic strain. By removing or modifying certain virulence genes, reverse genetics also can be used to convert highly pathogenic influenza viruses into vaccine candidates that are safer for vaccine manufacturers to handle.

Cell Culture

Another technique is use of cell cultures to grow vaccine strains; such as genetically engineering baculovirus to express a gene that encodes an influenza coat protein such as hemagglutinin or neuraminidase. "A recent NIAID-supported Phase II clinical trial of a vaccine produced by Protein Sciences Corporation using this strategy showed that it is well tolerated and immunogenic; the company is conducting further clinical evaluation of this product. Other new pathways for producing influenza vaccines include DNA-based approaches and the development of broadly protective vaccines based on influenza virus proteins that are shared by multiple strains."

AVI Bio Pharma Inc. has evidence of inhibition of multiple subtypes of influenza A virus in cell culture with Morpholino oligomers from the results of their labs and four independent research laboratories. "The key finding here is that our NEUGENE(R) therapeutics continue to show efficacy against all strains of influenza A, including H5N1." Morpholinos conjugated with cell penetrating peptides have been shown effective in protecting mice from influenza A.

"Several companies are focusing on new vehicles for growing antigens, which are the bits of a virus or bacterium needed to spur a person's immune system to fight an infection. VaxInnate, a New Jersey-based biotechnology company, has reported success using E. coli bacteria, which can cause a sometimes-fatal infection but also can be used to grow vaccine ingredients when the harmful part of the bacterium is removed. Dowpharma, a unit of Dow Chemical, has been using different bacteria found in soil and water, P. fluorescens, which may make a higher volume of antigens more quickly than E. coli." A recent study has shown promise by a vaccine called FluBlOk, which is made in insect cells. This experimental vaccine, which focuses on hemagglutinin, would cut the production process by one to two months, as well as avoiding other pitfalls of chicken eggs.

"The Committee for Medicinal Products for Human Use (CHMP), which reviews applications for 27 EU countries, found that Novartis's Optaflu vaccine, given to more than 3,400 people during clinical studies, met the CHMP's immunogenicity criteria [...] Novartis has said that Optaflu is a subunit vaccine, meaning it contains individual viral proteins rather than whole virus particles. [...] Novartis said it anticipates applying for US licensing of its cell-based flu vaccine in 2008. The company has conducted phase 1 and 2 clinical trials of the vaccine in the United States and in July 2006 announced it would build a $600 million plant in Holly Springs, N.C., to make cell-culture flu vaccines. In May 2006 the US Department of Health and Human Services awarded Novartis a $220 million contract to develop cell-based flu vaccines, and Novartis has said the money would go towards the cost of the new facility.

Depending on when its vaccine is approved by the Food and Drug Administration, the plant could begin production as early as 2011 and be ready for full production as early as 2012, with an annual output of 50 million doses of a trivalent vaccine, the company has said.

In the event of a flu pandemic, the facility is designed to have the capacity to make up to 150 million monovalent (single strain) doses each year within 6 months of a pandemic declaration, Novartis said. Novartis' other cell-based vaccine production facility is in Marburg, Germany."

H5N1 Vaccine Research

There are several H5N1 vaccines for several of the avian H5N1 varieties. H5N1 continually mutates rendering them, so far for humans, of little use. While there can be some cross-protection against related flu strains, the best protection would be from a vaccine specifically produced for any future pandemic flu virus strain. Dr. Daniel Lucey, co-director of the Biohazardous Threats and Emerging Diseases graduate programme at Georgetown University has made this point, "There is no H5N1 pandemic so there can be no pandemic vaccine." However, "pre-pandemic vaccines" have been created; are being refined and tested; and do have some promise both in furthering research and preparedness for the next pandemic. Vaccine manufacturing companies are being encouraged to increase capacity so that if a pandemic vaccine is needed, facilities will be available for rapid production of large amounts of a vaccine specific to a new pandemic strain.

Problems with H5N1 vaccine production include:

- lack of overall production capacity.
- lack of surge production capacity (it is impractical to develop a system that depends on hundreds of millions of 11-day old specialised eggs on a standby basis).
- the pandemic H5N1 might be lethal to chickens.

Cell culture (cell-based) manufacturing technology can be applied to influenza vaccines as they are with most viral vaccines and thereby solve the problems associated with creating flu vaccines using chicken eggs as is currently done. Researchers at the University of Pittsburgh have had success with a genetically engineered vaccine that took only a month to make and completely protected chickens from the highly pathogenic H5N1 virus.

According to the United States Department of Health and Human Services:

In addition to supporting basic research on cell-based influenza vaccine development, HHS is currently supporting a number of vaccine manufacturers in the advanced development of cell-based influenza vaccines with the goal of developing US-licensed cell-based influenza vaccines produced in the United States. Dose-sparing technologies. Current US-licensed vaccines stimulate an immune response based on the quantity of HA (hemagglutinin) antigen included in the dose. Methods to stimulate a strong immune response using less HA antigen are being studied in H5N1 and H9N2 vaccine trials. These include changing the mode of delivery from intramuscular to intradermal and the addition of immune-enhancing adjuvant to the vaccine formulation. Additionally, HHS is soliciting contract proposals from manufacturers of vaccines, adjuvants, and medical devices for the development and licensure of influenza vaccines that will provide dose-sparing alternative strategies.

Chiron Corporation is now recertified and under contract with the National Institutes of Health to produce 8,000-10,000 investigational doses of Avian Flu (H5N1) vaccine. Aventis Pasteur is under similar contract. The United States government hopes to obtain enough vaccine in 2006 to treat 4 million people. However, it is unclear whether this vaccine would be effective against a hypothetical mutated strain that would be easily transmitted through human populations, and the shelflife of stockpiled doses has yet to be determined.

The New England Journal of Medicine reported on March 30, 2006 on one of dozens of vaccine studies currently being conducted. The Treanor *et al.* study was on vaccine produced from the human isolate (A/Vietnam/1203/2004 H5N1) of a virulent clade 1 influenza A (H5N1) virus with the use of a plasmid rescue system, with only the hemagglutinin and neuraminidase genes expressed and administered without adjuvant. "The rest of the genes were derived from an avirulent egg-adapted influenza A/PR/8/34 strain.

The hemagglutinin gene was further modified to replace six basic amino acids associated with high pathogenicity in birds at the cleavage site between hemagglutinin 1 and hemagglutinin 2. Immunogenicity was assessed by microneutralisation and hemagglutination-inhibition assays with the use of the vaccine virus, although a subgroup of samples were tested with the use of the wild-type influenza A/Vietnam/1203/2004 (H5N1) virus." The results of this study combined with others scheduled to be completed by Spring 2007 is hoped will provide a highly immunogenic vaccine that is cross-protective against heterologous influenza strains.

H5N1 Vaccine Approval and Stockpiling

On April 17, 2007, the first US approval for H5N1 influenza vaccine for humans was given. This vaccine made by Sanofi-Aventis at a plant in Swiftwater, Pennsylvania is not to be sold commercially; instead the US is stockpiling it as an interim measure while better vaccines are being researched.

Two injections given 28 days apart gave evidence of providing protection for 45 per cent of the people who got the vaccine in a study. "The US Department of Health and Human Services said it had already purchased 13 million doses of the Sanofi vaccine, enough to inoculate 6.5 million people. The vaccine was approved for people age 18 to 64. Studies in other age groups are ongoing. The most common side effects reported were pain at the injection site, headache, general ill feeling and muscle pain, the FDA said."

This April 17, 2007 "approval by the Food and Drug Administration means the vaccine is no longer considered experimental and therefore could be dispensed during a pandemic without requiring each recipient to sign a form giving informed consent. The two injections combined contain 180 micrograms of antigen, the piece of the H5N1 virus designed to spur immunity. By contrast, a conventional flu shot contains 45 micrograms of antigen: 15 micrograms for each of the three strains it protects against."

The vaccine approved on April 17, 2007 "is based on an H5N1 virus isolated from a Vietnamese patient in 2004. Today's approval by the FDA follows a Feb. 27 recommendation by an FDA advisory panel, which found that the vaccine was safe and effective. However, some of the panel members had reservations about the immunogenicity of the vaccine, which in data submitted to the panel was somewhat lower than previously reported in a 2006 article in the New England Journal of Medicine. In a clinical trial, two 90-microgram (mcg) doses of the vaccine, administered to 103 healthy adults 28 days apart, generated a protective immune response in 45 per cent of recipients, the FDA noted. (The researchers used a neutralising antibody titer of 1:40, a fourfold or more increase in antibody titer, to define adequate immune response). The national stockpile currently contains 13 million doses of the H5N1 vaccine, enough to vaccinate 6.5 million people. HHS has said it is moving forward with the development of a "clade 2" H5N1 vaccine, based on viruses that circulated in birds in China and Indonesia in 2003-04 and spread to the Middle East, Europe, and Africa in 2005 and 2006."

13

Economic Impact

Influenza produces direct costs due to lost productivity and associated medical treatment, as well as indirect costs of preventative measures. In the United States, influenza is responsible for a total cost of over $10 billion per year, while it has been estimated that a future pandemic could cause hundreds of billions of dollars in direct and indirect costs.

However, the economic impacts of past pandemics have not been intensively studied, and some authors have suggested that the Spanish influenza actually had a positive long-term effect on per-capita income growth, despite a large reduction in the working population and severe short-term depressive effects. Other studies have attempted to predict the costs of a pandemic as serious as the 1918 Spanish flu on the US economy, where 30 per cent of all workers became ill, and 2.5 per cent were killed. A 30 per cent sickness rate and a three-week length of illness would decrease the gross domestic product by 5 per cent. Additional costs would come from medical treatment of 18 million to 45 million people, and total economic costs would be approximately $700 billion.

Preventative costs are also high. Governments worldwide have spent billions of US dollars preparing and planning for a potential H5N1 avian influenza pandemic, with costs associated with purchasing drugs and vaccines as well as developing disaster drills and strategies for improved border controls. On 1 November 2005, United States President George W. Bush unveiled the National Strategy to Safeguard Against the Danger of Pandemic Influenza backed by a request to Congress for $7.1 billion to begin implementing the plan. Internationally, on 18 January 2006, donor nations pledged US $2 billion to combat bird flu at the two-day International Pledging Conference on Avian and Human Influenza held in China.

Swine Flu Outbreak 2009

The 2009 swine flu outbreak is an epidemic of a new strain of Influenza A virus subtype H1N1 identified in April 2009. It is thought to be a mutation (reassortment) of four known strains of influenza A virus subtype H1N1: one endemic in humans, one endemic in birds, and two endemic in pigs (swine). A June 5th update by the UN's World Health Organisation (WHO) states that "69 countries have officially reported 21,940 cases of influenza A(H1N1) infection, including 125 deaths."

The outbreak began in Mexico, where early reports indicated a surge of cases that had already killed at least 81 people by April 26. As a result, WHO and the US Centres for Disease Control and Prevention (CDC) expressed concern that this could become a worldwide flu pandemic, with WHO raising its alert level to Phase 5 out of the six maximum, indicating that a flu pandemic is "imminent".

Most cases throughout the world have so far been mild relative to seasonal flu. But because this is a new virus, most people do not have immunity to it, and illness may eventually become more severe and widespread in different demographic and population groups.

This new H1N1 flu mainly spreads in humans in the same way that regular seasonal influenza spreads, which is through the air from coughs and sneezes or touching those infected. It cannot be transmitted from eating properly cooked pork.

There was no vaccine available to prevent infection as of June 2009, although companies were developing one for availability in late-July or August. There is concern that the virus could mutate over the coming months to a more dangerous flu outbreak later in the year, and a vaccine produced now might be less effective in preventing its spread.

Health officials in the US pointed out that the "terrible experience" of the 1918 flu pandemic, which killed approximately 600,000 in the United States alone, was preceded by a mild "herald" wave of cases in the spring.

As of May 24, nearly 90 per cent of reported deaths had taken place in Mexico. This led to speculation that Mexico may have been in the midst of an unrecognised epidemic for months prior to the current outbreak, thereby showing a fatality rate that was much higher than it would have been if earlier cases had been counted. According to the CDC, the fact that the flu's infection activity is now monitored more closely may also help explain why more flu cases than normal are being recorded in many countries.

Historical Context

Annual influenza epidemics are estimated to affect 5-15 per cent of the global population, resulting in severe illness in 3–5 million patients and causing 250,000-500,000 deaths worldwide. In industrialised countries severe illness and deaths occur mainly in the high-risk populations of infants, the elderly, and chronically ill patients.

In addition to these annual epidemics, Influenza A virus strains caused three major global pandemics during the 20th century: the Spanish flu in 1918, Asian flu in 1957 and Hong Kong flu in 1968-69. These pandemics were caused by strains of Influenza A virus that had undergone major genetic changes and for which the population did not possess significant immunity. The overall effects of these pandemics are summarised in the table below.

Flu Pandemics Over Last 100 Years

Pandemic	*Year*	*Influenza A virus subtype*	*People infected (approx.)*	*Deaths (est.)*	*Case fatality rate*
Spanish flu	1918–19	H1N1	1 billion	50 million	>5%
Asian flu	1957	H2N2		2 million	<0.1%
Hong Kong flu	1968–69	H3N2		1 million	<0.1%

The influenza virus has also caused several pandemic threats over the past century, including the pseudo-pandemic of 1947, the 1976 swine flu outbreak and the 1977 Russian flu, all caused by the H1N1 subtype. The world has been at an increased level of alert since the SARS epidemic in South East Asia (caused by the SARS coronavirus). The level of preparedness was further increased and sustained with the advent of the H5N1 bird flu outbreaks because of H5N1's high fatality rate, although the strains currently prevalent have limited human-to-human transmission (anthroponotic) capability, or epidemicity.

People who contracted flu prior to 1957 may have some immunity. A May 20 New York Times article stated: "Tests on blood serum from older people showed that they had antibodies that attacked the new virus, Dr. Daniel Jernigan, chief flu epidemiologist at the Centres for Disease Control and Prevention, said in a telephone news conference. That does not mean that everyone over 52 is immune, since some Americans and Mexicans older than that have died of the new flu."

Initial Outbreaks

This article covers the chronology of the 2009 novel influenza A (H1N1) epidemic. Flag icons denote the first announcements of confirmed cases by the respective nation-states, their first deaths (and other major events such as their first intergenerational cases and their first cases of zoonosis), and relevant sessions and announcements of the World Health Organisation, European Union, and the US Centres for Disease Control.

Unless otherwise noted, references to terms like S-OIV, H1N1 and such, all refer to this new A(H1N1) strain and not to sundry other strains of H1N1 which are endemic in humans, birds and pigs.

Timeline

March 2009: *Mexico:* In La Gloria, Veracruz, 60 per cent of the town's population is sickened by a respiratory illness of unknown provenance.

March 17: *Mexico:* Earliest known onset of a case that is later to be confirmed as Swine-Origin Influenza A (H1N1) Virus Infection.

March 18: *Mexico:* Surveillance begins picking up a surge in cases of influenza-like illness (ILI).

March 28: *United States:* Earliest known onset of a USA case later confirmed as swine flu, being a nine-year-old girl residing in Imperial County, California.

March 30: *United States:* Biosurveillance firm Veratect begins tracking the unusual respiratory illness in Mexico.

- *United States:* A sample is collected from a nine-year-old female patient which is later confirmed to contain the novel virus strain [genetically sequenced as A/ California/05/2009(H1N1)].
- *United States:* Onset of illness for a ten-year-old boy residing in San Diego County, California; his case is eventually the first to be confirmed as swine flu, .

April 2009:

April 1:

- *United States:* A nasopharyngeal swab is collected from a ten-year-old male patient in San Diego County, later confirmed as containing the novel virus and the first organism of that strain to be completely sequenced [A/ California/04/2009(H1N1)].

April 2:

- *Mexico:* In La Gloria, Veracruz, a four-year-old boy falls ill at the end of the outbreak. Only his sample, which was eventually sent abroad, tested positive for A(H1N1). Veracruz officials state that there were no plans to exhume the bodies of two infants who died in the outbreak.

April 6:

- *Mexico:* Public health authorities begin investigating unusual cases of pneumonia. 400 people had reportedly sought treatment for pneumonia/influenza-like illness (ILI) in La Gloria the preceding week.
- *United States:* Veratect publishes the alert "La Gloria: 'Strange' Respiratory Affects 60 per cent of Local Population; Three Paediatric Deaths May be Associated with the Outbreak."

April 12:

- *Mexico:* The General Directorate of Epidemiology (DGE) reports the outbreak of an ILI in a small community in Veracruz to the Pan American Health Organisation (PAHO), which is the Regional Office of the World Health Organisation (WHO).
- *Mexico:* A 39-year-old woman dies of severe viral pneumonia in the city of San Luis Potosi; this is later believed to be the earliest known fatality related to the outbreak.

April 13:

- *Mexico:* First death in Oaxaca due to what would later be identified as swine flu.
- *United States:* The Centres for Disease Control (CDC) is advised of a ten-year-old boy with a respiratory illness in San Diego County, California. Test results had revealed an Influenza A virus, but were negative for standard human strains. The San Diego County Health Department is notified.

April 14: *United States:* The CDC receives its first sample from California (from the ten-year-old boy in San Diego County), and identifies the virus as a strain of swine influenza A(H1N1).

April 16:

- *Mexico:* Authorities notify the PAHO of the atypical pneumonia.
- *United States:* Veratect publishes the alert "Atypical Pneumonia Cases Reported at Hospital" regarding the Oaxaca cases.

April 17: *United States:* The CDC receives a second sample from Southern California (taken from the nine-year-old girl in Imperial County), and again identifies the virus as a strain of swine influenza A(H1N1). The California Department of Public Health is notified.

- *Mexico:* A case of atypical pneumonia in Oaxaca prompts enhanced national surveillance. A field investigation is started. Mexico contacts Canada to request more specialised testing.

April 18: *Mexico:* Mexico sends 14 mucus samples to the CDC and dispatches health teams hospitals to look for patients showing severe influenza- or pneumonia-like symptoms.

April 20: *United States:* Veratect advises the CDC of the Mexican events. The CDC is already investigating the California and Texas cases.

April 21: *United States:* The CDC alerts physicians to a similar novel strain of swine influenza A(H1N1) in two cases from Southern California. Local investigations, including investigations in Texas, are underway, and overall surveillance is enhanced. The Associated Press covers the alert, the first mention of the A(H1N1) outbreak in English-language media.

April 22: *Canada:* Canada receives samples from Mexico for testing.

April 23: *Mexico:* The Public Health Agency of Canada confirms Mexico cases of swine-origin influenza A (H1N1) virus (S-OIV) infection. Genetic sequence analysis reveals that the Mexican patients were infected with the same S-OIV strain detected in two California children. The PAHO is informed that a cluster in Mexico of severe respiratory illnesses has been laboratory-confirmed as S-OIV infection.

April 24: The WHO issues its first Disease Outbreak Notice on the matter, confirming the infection of a number of people in Mexico and the United States by "Swine Influenza A/H1N1 viruses... not... previously detected in pigs or humans."

- *United States:* The CDC tells a press conference that seven of the 14 Mexican samples contained the same virus strain as the known in California and Texas, and that indications suggested that containment in the USA was "not very likely".
- *Mexico:* The Minister of Health confirms the Mexican cases of human infection by swine influenza and states that it believes that some of these cases had resulted in death. Health authorities implement public health measures for all airport passengers and the vaccination of health care workers with seasonal influenza vaccine.

April 25: WHO Under the International Health Regulations (IHR), the newly convened Emergency Committee meets for the first time, resulting in the WHO Director-General declaring a formal "public health emergency of international concern".

The PAHO Vaccination Week In The Americas starts. The 2009 Week was planned to emphasise the vaccination of entire families, and health worker immunisation.

- *United States:* First closure of an entire school district, the Schertz-Cibolo-Universal City Independent School District outside San Antonio, Texas.

April 26-27: WHO The Emergency Committee meets for the second time. The WHO Director-General issues a statement that containment of the outbreak is not feasible, and elevates the pandemic alert from Phase 3 to Phase 4.

- *Canada:* First six cases confirmed, four in Nova Scotia and two in British Columbia.
- *Spain:* First confirmed case of swine flu, in Almansa, and thus the first case in Europe; A(H1N1) has spread from the WHO Region of the Americas to the WHO European Region.
- *United Kingdom:* First two confirmed cases, in Scotland.
- *European Union (EU):* Health Commissioner advises Europeans not to travel to the United States or Mexico unless the need is urgent. This follows the first confirmed case in Spain.
- *Mexico:* First seven confirmed deaths.

April 28: WHO Confirmed cases are now extant in four of six WHO regions. As of 1915 GMT seven countries have officially reported cases of swine influenza A(H1N1) infection.

- *Israel:* First confirmed case in Israel and thus the WHO Eastern Mediterranean Region (colour-coded yellow), the third region to be affected.
- *New Zealand:* First three confirmed cases in New Zealand and thus the WHO Western Pacific Region (colour-coded red), the fourth region to be affected.
- *Canada:* Confirmed: two cases and another four in Alberta and Ontario, respectively.
- *Spain:* The second confirmed case in Spain is located in Valencia.

April 29: WHO The Emergency Committee meets for the third time, and the WHO raises its pandemic alert level from Phase 4 to Phase 5, its second highest. As of 1800 GMT, nine countries have officially reported 148 cases of swine influenza A(H1N1) infection. EU Foreign Relations Commissioner Benita Ferrero-Waldner announces that the halt of all travel to Mexico and disinfecting all airports due to the global flu outbreak is being considered.

- *Germany:* First three confirmed cases, two in Bavaria and one in Hamburg.

- *Austria:* First confirmed case.
- *United States:* First death outside Mexico, a 23-month-old Mexican child hospitalised in Texas. Ninety-one cases confirmed cases worldwide to date.
- *Spain:* Eight more cases raises the total in Spain to 10, including the first human-to-human intergenerational transmission (in which the patient had not recently been to Mexico but was infected by another patient who had just visited Mexico, namely his girlfriend). This is the first intergenerational transmission to be documented in Europe.
- *Canada:* Nineteen confirmed cases.
- *United Kingdom:* Three more confirmed cases of swine flu, giving a total of five confirmed cases.

April 30: Netherlands First confirmed case, a three-year-old child. The child returned from Mexico to the Netherlands on April 27, 2009. The parents test negative for A(H1N1).

- *Switzerland:* First confirmed case.
- *Ireland:* First confirmed case.
- *United States:* Four cases are confirmed in an outbreak at the University of Delaware; another 12 cases are deemed "probable". One of the confirmed cases is a baseball player, which results in the university cancelling sporting events, a concert by rapper Young Jeezy, and other school activities.
- *Canada:* Confirmed One more case in Toronto, and eight more cases in Nova Scotia, and Alberta bringing total to 28.
- *United Kingdom:* Three further confirmed cases of swine flu, giving a total of eight confirmed cases.

May 2009:

May 1: WHO As of 0600 GMT, 11 countries have officially reported 331 cases of influenza A(H1N1) infection.

- Hong Kong, China:
  - — 300 people are placed under quarantine at a hotel for seven days due to Hong Kong's first confirmed case there.
  - — Chief Executive Donald Tsang raises Hong Kong's response level from "serious" to "emergency".
  - — The Director of Health, Dr. PY Lam, orders Metropark Hotel in Wan Chai to be isolated for 7 days.
- *Denmark:* First confirmed case (in Hvidovre).
- *France:* First two confirmed cases.
- *United Kingdom:* First and second case of human to human (or intergenerational) transmission within the UK confirmed.
- *United States:* 155 confirmed cases. Two confirmed cases at the George Washington University's Thurston Hall.
- *Canada:* 51 Confirmed Cases.
- *Mexico:* Begins five-day shutdown to fight flu spread.

May 2: WHO As of 0600 GMT 15 countries have officially reported 615 cases of influenza A(H1N1) infection.

- *Italy:* First confirmed case.
- *South Korea:* First confirmed case.
- *Costa Rica:* First confirmed case, and the first in Central America.
- *China:* Suspends flights from Mexico to Shanghai when a case is confirmed on a flight from Mexico.
- Canada:
  - — 85 confirmed cases.
  - — The Canadian Food Inspection Agency confirms the first human-to-animal transmission of the virus after an Albertan returns from Mexico and infects a pig farm, the first known case of (reverse) zoonosis.

- *Mexico:* The fatal and confirmed cases are corrected to 101 and 397, respectively.
- *United States:* 189 confirmed cases. There are more than 430 schools closures in 18 states.

May 3: WHO As of 0600 GMT, 17 countries have officially reported 787 cases of (A)H1N1.

- *Colombia:* First confirmed case in South America.
- *Portugal:* First confirmed case.
- *Mexico:* Final day of lock-down in Mexico.
- *Canada:* 101 confirmed cases after seven cases in British Columbia, three in Alberta, two in Nova Scotia and Ontario, and one in Quebec were confirmed.

May 4: WHO As of 06:00 GMT, 20 countries have officially reported 985 cases of influenza A (H1N1) infection.

- *El Salvador:* First confirmed case.
- *Israel:* Second confirmed case.
- *Canada:* A girl from Edmonton, Alberta was diagnosed with a severe case of the H1N1 virus, the first severe one in Canada.

May 5: WHO As of 06:00 GMT, 21 countries have officially reported 1,124 cases of influenza A (H1N1) infection.

- *Guatemala:* First confirmed case.
- United States:
  - — Second confirmed death, the first of a US resident, a pregnant special education teacher in Texas: Judy Trunnell. The 33-year-old gives birth to her second child via Caesarian section during her eighth month of pregnancy, in a coma whilst on life support. Judy Trunnell had several underlying medical conditions, most notably asthma.
  - — Several sailors in San Diego, California fall ill (including a sailor on the USS Dubuque, which results in the cancellation of its deployment). These are the first cases in the US Navy.

— As the low level of virulence of novel A(H1N1) in the US becomes established, the CDC issues revised criteria for school closures, effectively ending widespread shutdowns.

May 6: WHO As of 06:00 GMT, 22 countries have officially reported 1,516 cases of influenza A (H1N1) infection.

- *Poland:* First confirmed case.
- *Sweden:* First confirmed case.

May 7: WHO As of 18:00 GMT, 24 countries have officially reported 2371 cases of influenza A (H1N1) infection.

- *Argentina:* First confirmed case.
- *Brazil:* First four confirmed cases.
- *Canada:* Reports suggest that an elderly woman who had swine flu has died in northern Alberta, marking the first death in Canada related to swine flu.
- *The Netherlands:* A second and a third confirmed case has been reported, by a 53-year-old woman and a 52-year-old man.
- *USA:* The New England Journal of Medicine establishes its H1N1 Influenza Centre on its website.

May 8: WHO As of 16:00 GMT, 25 countries have officially reported 2,500 cases of influenza A (H1N1) infection.

- *Japan:* First three confirmed cases.
- *Panama:* First confirmed case.

May 9: WHO As of 06:00 GMT, 29 countries have officially reported 3,440 cases of influenza A(H1N1) infection.

- *Australia:* First confirmed case.
- *Brazil:* Two cases confirmed, one of which is thought to be the first case of human-to-human infection in Brazil.
- *Costa Rica:* First confirmed death, and also the first death outside of North America. Three other confirmed cases, all children, were contaminated by the patient who died.

- *Norway:* First two confirmed cases.
- *USA:* Third confirmed death, a Washington man with underlying heart disease. Also, the USA passes Mexico in the number of confirmed cases of infection, 1693 to 1364, thus becoming the nation-state with the most laboratory-confirmed cases of infection; Canada is third with 242 cases.

May 10: WHO As of 07:30 GMT, 29 countries have officially reported 4,379 cases of influenza A(H1N1) infection.

- *Sweden:* Second confirmed case.
- *China:* First confirmed case.
- *Brazil:* More two cases confirmed. Now the country has 8 confirmed cases.

May 11: WHO As of 06:00 GMT, 30 countries have officially reported 4,694 cases of influenza A(H1N1) infection.

May 12: WHO As of 06:00 GMT, 30 countries have officially reported 5,251 cases of influenza A(H1N1) infection.

- *Cuba:* First confirmed case.
- *Thailand:* First two confirmed cases. Thailand is the first South East Asia country to be affected by the virus.
- *Finland:* First two confirmed cases.
- *Brazil:* Beyond the eight confirmed cases, the country has 34 suspected cases.
- *Panama:* 11 new confirmed cases. 29 total.
- *Canada:* The first case in Yukon Territory is confirmed.
- *Spain:* 100 cases confirmed.

May 13: WHO As of 06:00 GMT, 13 May 2009, 33 countries have officially reported 5,728 cases of influenza A(H1N1) infection.

- *China:* Second confirmed case.
- *Hong Kong:* China Second confirmed case.
- *Belgium:* First confirmed case.

- *Panama:* 10 more cases confirmed today. Total :39.
- *Argentina:* Second confirmed case.

May 14: WHO As of 06:00 GMT, 33 countries have officially reported 6,497 cases of influenza A(H1N1) infection.

- *Belgium:* Second confirmed case.
- *Colombia:* First domestic infections with 3 cases confirmed. Total: 10.
- *Peru:* First confirmed case.

May 15: WHO As of 06:00 GMT, 34 countries have officially reported 7,520 cases of influenza A(H1N1) infection.

- *USA:* Fourth and fifth deaths confirmed, that of an Arizona woman suffering from a lung condition and a Texas man in Corpus Christi, respectively.
- *Malaysia:* First confirmed case. Malaysia is the 37th country to be affected by the virus.
- *Belgium:* 2 more cases confirmed today. Total: 4.
- *Ecuador:* First confirmed case.
- *Cuba:* 2 more cases confirmed today. Total: 3.
- *Panama:* 4 new cases confirmed today. Total: 43, 23 of whom are male and 20 of whom are female. 20 of the cases are under 15 years old.

May 16: WHO As of 06:00 GMT 36 countries have officially reported 8,451 cases of influenza A(H1N1) infection.

- *Malaysia:* Second confirmed case. The first patient is now showing significant improvement from the treatment.
- *Japan:* First domestic infection confirmed, in Kobe, a male high school student with no history of travel abroad. The Kobe Festival, planned for May 16 and 17, is cancelled.
- *India:* First case confirmed, in Hyderabad. This marks the arrival of A(H1N1) in the fifth of the WHO's six regions, the South-East Asia Region.

- *Turkey:* First confirmed case.
- *Panama:* 11 New confirmed cases. 54 total.

May 17: WHO As of 06:00 GMT 37 countries have officially reported 8,480 cases of influenza A(H1N1) infection.

- *Panama:* With 54 confirmed cases, Panama occupies second place, along with Canada, for the number of cases per country.
- *Chile:* First confirmed case in the country, and the 41st country affected.

May 18: WHO As of 06:00 GMT, 40 countries have officially reported 8,829 cases of influenza A(H1N1) infection, including 74 deaths.

- *USA:* The sixth death in the US, and the first in New York —that of an assistant principal.
- *Japan:* reports 96 confirmed cases; it now ranks fourth in the world in the number of infections. Thousands of schools in 21 cities in the Hyogo and Osaka prefectures are temporarily closed.
- *Greece:* First confirmed case.
- *United Kingdom:* 107 cases confirmed.

May 19: WHO As of 06:00 GMT, 40 countries have officially reported 9,830 cases of influenza A(H1N1) infection, including 79 deaths.

- *United States:* Seventh confirmed death, that of a 44-year-old Missouri man.
- *Japan:* 191 confirmed cases; Hyogo Prefecture has the most at 111.
- *Peru:* 2 more cases confirmed today. Total: 3.
- *Norway:* 1 more case confirmed today. Total: 3.
- *Paraguay:* confirmed its first case and became the 43rd affected country.
- *Taiwan:* Confirmed its first case and becomes the 44th affected country.

May 20: WHO As of 06:00 GMT, 40 countries have officially reported 10,243 cases of influenza A(H1N1) infection, including 80 deaths.

- *United States:* A patient dies in Arizona, and a 22-year-old man dies in Utah, the nation's eighth and ninth H1N1 fatalities. Roughly half of the influenza viruses detected by the CDC's routine influenza surveillance systems are now that of novel A(H1N1). An unusual number of outbreaks in schools is reported.
- *Japan:* 236 confirmed cases, including the first case in Shiga Prefecture, and Hachioji and Kawasaki city in the Greater Tokyo Area. Two female high school students from Tokyo who had recently attended a Model United Nations conference in New York are presumed to have become infected abroad.
- *Norway:* 1 more case confirmed today. Total: 4.
- *Brazil:* 1 more confirmed case, now are 9 cases in total.

May 21: WHO As of 06:00 GMT, 41 countries have officially reported 11,034 cases of influenza A(H1N1) infection, including 85 deaths.

- *Japan:* 279 confirmed cases; more than 4,800 schools are closed in the Kobe region.
- *Philippines:* Confirms first case of influenza A(H1N1) virus.

May 22: WHO As of 06:00 GMT, 42 countries have officially reported 11,168 cases of influenza A(H1N1) infection, including 86 deaths.

- *Japan:* 317 confirmed, including first confirmed in Saitama Prefecture. Third confirmed in Tokyo, a 25-year-old man who visited Osaka from May 14-20th.
- *Russia:* First confirmed case.
- *Honduras:* First confirmed case.

May 23: WHO As of 06:00 GMT, 43 countries have officially reported 12,022 cases of influenza A(H1N1) infection, including 86 deaths.

- *Iceland:* First confirmed case. 4 more cases suspected.
- *South Korea:* has six more confirmed cases. Total: 10
- *Chile:* 55 confirmed cases
- *United Kingdom:* 122 cases confirmed.
- *Brazil:* has one more confirmed case. Total: 10.

May 24: Kuwait First confirmed cases, that of 18 US soldiers.

- *Australia:* Two more confirmed cases, which now brings the national toll to 16.
- *Philippines:* Second confirmed case reported by Philippine Health secretary Francisco Duque.
- *United Kingdom:* 133 cases confirmed.
- *Argentina:* 3 cases confirmed. Total: 5
- *United Arab Emirates:* First case confirmed.

May 25: WHO As of 06:00 GMT, 46 countries have officially reported 12,515 cases of influenza A(H1N1) infection, including 91 deaths.

- *United Kingdom:* 4 more confirmed cases in the United Kingdom. Total: 137.
- *Canada:* Second confirmed death in Ontario.
- *Australia:* 22 Confirmed Cases.
- *Ireland:* Second confirmed case.
- *Bahrain:* First confirmed case.
- *United States:* 12th death confirmed.
- *Czech Republic:* First confirmed case

May 26: WHO As of 06:00 GMT, 46 countries have officially reported 12,954 cases of influenza A(H1N1) infection, including 92 deaths

- *Argentina:* 14 Confirmed Cases. Total: 19.
- *United Kingdom:* 44 new cases confirmed. Total: 184

- *Chile:* 107 confirmed cases.
- *Australia:* 61 confirmed cases.
- *Puerto Rico:* First confirmed case

May 27: WHO As of 06:00 GMT, 48 countries have officially reported 13,398 cases of influenza A(H1N1) infection, including 95 deaths.

- *Singapore:* First confirmed case. A 22-year-old woman picked up the virus after visiting New York.
- *Romania:* First confirmed case.
- *Philippines:* Four more confirmed cases.
- *Dominican Republic:* First two confirmed cases.
- *United Kingdom:* 2 new cases confirmed. Total: 186
- *Chile:* 46 new cases confirmed. Total: 165
- *Argentina:* 37 cases confirmed.
- *Uruguay:* Confirmed its first two cases of Influenza A (H1N1).
- *Greece:* Confirmed two more cases.
- *Brazil:* has one more confirmed case. Total: 11

May 28:

- *Australia:* 147 Confirmed Cases.
- *Slovakia:* First confirmed case.
- *Singapore:* Three more cases confirmed. Total confirmed cases now stands at four.
- *United Kingdom:* Seventeen more confirmed cases Total: 203.
- *Sweden:* One more confirmed case. Total: 4.
- *Argentina:* 70 cases confirmed.
- *Chile:* 199 cases confirmed.
- *Bolivia:* First 2 cases confirmed.
- *Venezuela:* First case confirmed.
- *Philippines:* 4 new cases.

- *Brazil:* Has 3 new cases, the both are in Sao Paulo. Now the country has 14 cases.

May 29: WHO As of 06:00 GMT, 53 countries have officially reported 15,510 cases of influenza A(H1N1) infection, including 99 deaths.

- *United Kingdom:* 14 confirmed cases. Total: 217.
- *Norway:* One new confirmed case. Total: 5.
- *Hungary:* First confirmed case.
- *Brazil:* Another one case confirmed, being the third case of human-to-human transmission inside the country. Total: 15.
- *Uruguay:* 4 new confirmed cases. Total: 6.
- *Greece:* Another one case confirmed. Total: 4.
- *Venezuela:* Second confirmed case.
- *Philippines:* Health officials confirmed additional 4 cases. Total: 14 cases.

May 30:

- *Sweden:* One more confirmed case. Total: 5.
- *Norway:* Two new confirmed cases. Total: 7.
- *United Kingdom:* 12 more cases. Total: 229.
- *Cyprus:* First confirmed case.
- *Estonia:* First confirmed case.
- *Brazil:* Five more cases. Total: 20 (15 outside the country and 5 inside the country).
- *Lebanon:* First three cases confirmed.
- *Philippines:* 2 more cases confirmed.

May 31:

- *Vietnam:* First case confirmed.
- *Antarctica:* First two cases confirmed in two American scientists stationed there.
- *Singapore:* Another confirmed case brings the total confirmed to 5.

- *Argentina:* 100 cases confirmed.
- *Dominican:* Republic Nine more cases confirmed, for a total of 11 cases nationwide.
- *Uruguay:* 11 cases confirmed.
- *United Kingdom:* 14 more cases confirmed Total: 244.
- *Bahamas:* First confirmed case.

June 2009:

June 1: WHO As of 06:00 GMT, 62 countries have officially reported 17,410 cases of influenza A(H1N1) infection, including 115 deaths.

- *Philippines:* Additional 5 confirmed cases of A(H1N1) virus, in total of 21 confirmed case.
- *Australia:* Total: 401 cases.
- *Romania:* 5 confirmed cases.
- *Greece:* One more case confirmed total: 5.
- *Singapore:* Another two new confirmed cases. Total: 7 cases.
- *Bulgaria:* First confirmed case.
- *Israel:* 7 cases confirmed Total: 33.
- *United States:* West Virginia is the last USA state to be affected by swine flu.
- *Honduras:* 2 more cases confirmed Total: 3.
- *Canada:* 3rd death confirmed. First death in Toronto.
- *Venezuela:* Third confirmed case.

June 2:

- *Luxembourg:* First case confirmed.
- *Thailand:* 1 new confirmed case in total of 5 positive cases of A(H1N1) virus.
- *Ukraine:* First confirmed case of A (H1N1) virus.
- *Singapore:* One more confirmed case. Total: 8.
- *Egypt:* First confirmed case of A (H1N1) virus. First confirmed case in Africa.

- *Nicaragua:* First confirmed case of A (H1N1) virus.
- *Dominican Republic:* Two more cases of A (H1N1) virus. Total confirmed: 14.
- *United Kingdom:* New cases brings total to 339.
- *Sweden:* One more confirmed case. Total: 7.
- *Chile:* First confirmed death, a 37-year-old man.
- *Honduras:* 34 confirmed cases in total.
- *Bermuda:* First case confirmed.
- *Netherlands:* 1 more case confirmed. Total: 4.
- *Brazil:* 3 more case confirmed. Total: 23.

June 3: WHO As of 06:00 GMT, 3 June 2009, 66 countries have officially reported 19,273 cases of influenza A(H1N1) infection, including 117 deaths.

- *Saudi Arabia:* First case confirmed.
- *Philippines:* 1 new confirmed case in total of 22 positive cases of A(H1N1) virus.
- *Norway:* One new confirmed case. Total: 8.
- *Singapore:* Three new confirmed cases. Total: 11.
- *United Kingdom:* More Confirmed cases. Total: 404.
- *Venezuela:* 4th confirmed case.
- *Dominican Republic:* Total amount of confirmed cases rises to 23.
- *Nicaragua:* 4 new confirmed cases. Total: 5.
- *Barbados:* First case confirmed.
- *Jamaica:* First 2 cases confirmed.
- *New Zealand:* One further confirmed case, bringing the national total to 11.
- *Brazil:* 2 more cases confirmed. Total: 25.

June 4:

- *Philippines:* Confirmed cases of A(H1N1) virus rose to 29.

- *Malaysia:* Three more cases confirmed. One of the patient is a 23-year-old student returned from United States. Another two patients are German tourists who arrived in Singapore but went to Malaysia for holiday. Total: 5.
- *Norway:* One new confirmed case. Total: 9.
- *Sweden:* First domestic infection. Total: 13 (1 domestic).
- *United States:* The USA report another death in Connecticut, bringing the total up to 29.
- *Peru:* 49 confirmed cases of influenza A in Peru.
- *Guatemala:* 23 confirmed cases of influenza A in Guatemala.
- *Colombia:* 24 confirmed cases of influenza A in Colombia.
- *Brazil:* 3 more cases confirmed. Total: 28.
- *Singapore:* 12th case confirmed.
- *Panama:* Cases of influenza A is increased from 155 to 179 in Panama.
- *El Salvador:* Cases of influenza A infection in El Salvador increased to 49.
- *Austria:* 4 confirmed cases in Austria.
- *Trinidad and Tobago:* First case reported in the country.
- *Uruguay:* 17 cases reported in the country.
- *Ecuador:* 47 cases reported in the country.
- *Nicaragua:* 12 cases reported in the country.
- *Argentina:* 163 cases of influenza A in Argentina.
- *New Zealand:* 2 new confirmed cases, bringing the national total to 13.

June 5:

WHO As of 06:00 GMT, 69 countries have officially reported 21,940 cases of influenza A(H1N1) infection, including 125 deaths.

- *Malaysia:* Sixth case confirmed.
- *Philippines:* Four new confirmed cases. Total: 33.

- *Bulgaria:* Second case confirmed, a 7-year old from Blagoevgrad. Total: 2.
- *Cayman Islands:* First case confirmed.
- *Singapore:* Two new confirmed cases. Total: 14.
- *Spain:* 291 confirmed cases total in the country.
- *Ecuador:* 51 confirmed cases in the country.
- *Australia:* Australia now over the 1000 cases. Total: 1006.
- *Dominican Republic:* First fatality, a 17-year-old pregnant girl. Total amount of confirmed cases rises to 44.
- *Sweden:* One new domestic infection. Total: 14 (2 domestic).
- *Brazil 3:* More confirmed cases. Total: 31.

June 6:

- *Malaysia:* One more case confirmed. Total: 7.
- *Singapore:* One more case confirmed, which happens to be a local case. Total: 15.
- *Brazil:* 4 more confirmed cases. Total: 35.

June 7:

- *China:* Five more cases confirmed. Total: 72.
- *South Korea:* One more case confirmed. Total: 47.
- *New Zealand:* Authorities have confirmed that a man travelling from North America has Influenza A(H1N1). Total: 14.
- *Cuba:* Cuba confirmed fifth case of influenza A (H1N1).
- *Chile:* Chilean authorities confirms second death from influenza A in South America.
- *Venezuela:* 3 new cases in the country. Total: 7.
- *Brazil:* 1 new case in the country. Total: 36.

June 8:

WHO As of 06:00 GMT, 73 countries have officially reported 25,288 cases of influenza A(H1N1) infection, including 139 deaths.

- *New Zealand:* Three more confirmed cases, two of which were from international flights. Total: 17.
- *Philippines:* Thirteen more confirmed cases. Total: 46.
- *Sweden:* Two more domestic confirmed cases. Total: 16 (4 domestic).
- *Netherlands:* Ten more confirmed cases including two human-to-human infections. Total: 20.
- *Venezuela:* 5 new infections. Total: 12.
- *Dominican Republic:* Total amount of confirmed cases rises to 72.
- *Honduras:* 67 cases of influenza A H1N1 in Honduras.
- *Costa Rica:* Government confirms 93 positive cases of influenza A in Costa Rica.

June 9:

- *Singapore:* Two more confirmed case.
- Mexico.

The outbreak was first detected in Mexico City on March 18, where surveillance began picking up a surge in cases of influenza-like illness. The surge was initially assumed by Mexican authorities to be "late-season flu" outbreak and not a new virus strain. Health Secretary Jose Angel Cordova confirmed that a 4-year-old boy was part of an outbreak in Veracruz state that began in February. Residents of the town of Perote worried at the time that they had contracted a new and aggressive flu, and publicly demonstrated against the pig farm they initially blamed for their illness. It was only after US labs confirmed a swine flu outbreak that Mexican officials sent the boy's sample in for testing, and it tested positive for swine flu. While there was speculation that the outbreak may have started at the pig plant in Veracruz, the plant owners said that no pigs had tested positive for the virus.

After the outbreak was officially announced, Mexico immediately requested material support from the US and worked closely with the CDC and Canada, sending them suspected samples for testing. Soon after, the CDC helped Mexico build their own lab capability to do faster diagnosis and confirmation of the H1N1 virus in Mexico. According to one commentator, "in the face of mounting hysteria, the response of both Mexico and the United States was an almost perfect display of the cooperation and partnership . . . ." Within a few days Mexico City was "effectively shut down," and some countries hastily cancelled flights to Mexico while other halted trade. Although many in the US called for shutting the border to help contain the spread, President Obama rejected the idea and Homeland Security Secretary Janet Napolitano called it "pointless," as the virus had already crossed into the US, and felt that "closing the border would have done nothing more than wreak economic havoc on both economies."

As the outbreak spread throughout Mexico and into the US, however, scientists were trying to understand why there were so many deaths in Mexico while infections in the United States and Canada were relatively mild and not unusually dangerous compared to seasonal flue. "If that continues to be true," wrote the *Washington Post*, "then it may help explain the mysteriously high mortality in Mexico." The newspaper noted that "it may be that Mexico already has had hundreds of thousands, and possibly millions, of cases — all but the most serious hidden in the 'noise' of background illness in a crowded population." They added, "the fact that most people infected in other countries had recently been to Mexico — or were in direct contact with someone who had been — is indirect evidence that the country may have been experiencing a silent epidemic for months." A study published May 11 in the journal *Science* estimated Mexico alone may have already had 23,000 cases of swine flu by April 23, the day it announced the epidemic.

As experts struggled to explain why so many deaths had initially occurred in Mexico and nowhere else, the CDC on May 1, suggested a simple explanation: "there are many cases in Mexico, most are mild, and just the bad ones have been seen so far." It noted that recent severe cases had focused on patients seeking care in hospitals and acknowledged that there could in fact be a large number of undetected cases of illness, which would explain the much higher mortality rate. Other experts agreed: "The central question every flu expert in the world would like answered, is how many mild cases Mexico has had," said Dr. Martin Cetron, director of global migration and quarantine for the Centres for Disease Control, in an interview. "We may just be looking at the tip of the iceberg, which would give you a skewed initial estimate of the case fatality rate," as he also speculated that there may have been tens of thousands of unreported mild infections, which would then make the number of deaths seemingly low, and as the flu spreads, the number of people who become seriously ill would remain relatively small.

United States: Further information: 2009 swine flu outbreak in the United States

The place the virus originated is unknown. Analysis has suggested that the H1N1 strain responsible for the current outbreak first evolved around September 2008 and circulated in the human population for several months before the first cases were detected. The new strain was first diagnosed in two children by the CDC, first on April 14 in San Diego County, California and a few days later in nearby Imperial County, California. Neither child had been in contact with pigs.

World Governments and Media Response

US Response Analysed: According to Dr. Thomas Frieden, the new CDC director as of June 8, 2009: "There's no question that a new strain of influenza spreading rapidly throughout the world is a major problem and requires a major response. So far, it doesn't seem to be any more severe than seasonal flu, but seasonal flu kills 36,000 Americans a year."

Federal officials and other groups felt that six years of worrying about H5N1 avian flu did much to prepare the United States for the current swine flu outbreak. Jeffrey Levi, executive director of the monitoring group Trust for America's Health, notes that after H5N1 emerged widely in Asia in 2003, killing about 60 per cent of the humans infected by it, many countries took steps to prevent any crisis that would emerge if that virus were to acquire the ability to jump easily from human to human, and the measures taken in preparation were helpful. Levi also said that little vaccine would be available by the fall, even if there were no major delays in production.

Dr. Schuchat, summarising much of the country's quick response says "This really was a wake-up call for the world. We actually have been preparing for a pandemic for many years now." The avian flu outbreak more than five years ago led the CDC and state and local public health departments to prepare for a nationwide pandemic. "I would say these exercises worked immensely," Schuchat said, especially development of disease diagnosis and tracking and communication. "There has been a lot of payoff for worrying about bird flu."

But recognising that the responses were not perfect, she also said the CDC will now use the current lull to take stock of the nation's response to the new H1N1 flu and attempt to patch any gaps in the public health safety net before flu season starts this fall. She cited a new report which found that recent cuts in public health departments have meant many did not have adequate resources to carry out flu plans. The US Government Accountability Office also said the US flu preparedness plan needed improvement, including better coordination between federal, state and local governments and the private sector.

The report found problems in plans for school closings and limiting mass gatherings, and even with a mild outbreak, it found hospital emergency departments and other parts of the health care delivery system were overwhelmed. It urged government health officials to improve coordination at all levels of government and with other countries, and develop better strategies for school closings, sick-leave policies and other ways to limit public gatherings during periods of rapid infection. The report specifically urged a halt to planned layoffs at state and local health departments, and recommended hospitals improve strategies for handling a large influx of patients.

Data Accuracy

The initial outbreak received a week of near-constant media attention. Epidemiologists cautioned that the number of cases reported in the early days of an outbreak can be very inaccurate and deceptive due to several causes, among them selection bias, media bias, and incorrect reporting by governments. Inaccuracies could also be caused by authorities in different countries looking at differing population groups. Poverty may in part explain higher mortality rates in Mexico. Furthermore, countries with poor health care systems and older laboratory facilities may take longer to identify or report cases.

In late-April, experts predicted there would be 2,000 to 2,500 US cases by the end of May. However, by May 15, the Centres for Disease Control and Prevention estimated that there were "upwards of 100,000" cases in the country, even though only 7,415 had been confirmed at that point. Tim Germann, a computational scientist who worked on a 2006 flu forecast model at Los Alamos National Laboratory, has estimated there were now "a few hundred thousand" cases. The CDC and state health departments were reported to have stopped confirming most cases in laboratories.

In some instances, governments accused other countries of intentionally underreporting cases. Moscow, for instance, hinted that the Caribbean nation of the Dominican Republic was underreporting its number of swine flu cases to "boost tourism," and on May 30 advised its citizens not to travel there. In early-May, Cuba's Fidel Castro accused Mexico of hiding the scope of the epidemic until after President Obama visited the country in April, and a study published in the journal *Science* on May 11, estimated Mexico alone may have had 23,000 cases of swine flu by April 23, the day it announced the epidemic.

In the US data accuracy has also become an issue, with some school districts deciding to keep the names of students and schools that have reported infections confidential, one stating that "it would not be fair to single out one school," since doing so would likely trigger requests by parents to have their children tested despite their health not being in danger, and the schools lack the ability to test everyone. Dr. Hector Gonzalez Director of the Laredo Health Department said that according to CDC guidelines, physicians only need to submit samples for testing if the patient is a child under 5 years of age, is pregnant, has an underlying medical condition or is suffering from respiratory distress requiring urgent care.

Travel Advisories

The new strain has spread widely beyond Mexico and the US, with confirmed cases in fifty-four countries and suspected cases in fifty-nine. Many countries had earlier advised citizens to avoid travelling to infected areas, especially Mexico, and were monitoring visitors returning from flu-affected areas for possible flu symptoms. In late-April Mexico closed all of its schools and public places for a week to control its spread.

At first, most cases outside North America were recent travellers to Mexico or the US. However, intra-national infections have now also been reported from Canada, Japan, Panama, the UK, Spain, Germany, Australia, Italy, and Belgium.

On May 15, CDC's "Travel Health Warning" recommending against non-essential travel to Mexico, in effect since April 27, was downgraded to a "Travel Health Precaution for Mexico." In lifting its warning, the CDC said, "There is evidence that the Mexican outbreak is slowing down in many cities though not all." It also said that the "risk of severe disease" from the H1N1 virus "now appears to be less than originally thought."

Airline Hygiene Precautions

US airlines have made no major changes as of the beginning of June, but continued standing practices that include looking for passengers with symptoms of flu, measles or other infections, and rely on in-flight air filters to ensure that aircraft are sanitised. "We take our guidance from the professionals (such as the CDC)", stated an Air Transport Association spokesman. The CDC has not recommended that airline crews wear face masks or disposable overcoats.

Outside the US however, some airlines have modified hygiene procedures to minimise travel health risks on international flights. Asian carriers have stepped up cabin cleaning, installed state-of-the-art air filters and allowed in-flight staff to wear face masks, with some replacing used pillows, blankets, headset covers and headrest covers, while others have begun disinfecting the cabins of all aircraft. In China, some airline flight attendants are required to wear disposable facial masks, gloves and hats and even disposable overcoats during flights to select destinations.

Singapore has been thermal-screening everyone coming into the country, with Singapore Airlines giving passengers travelling to the United States health kits that include a thermometer, masks and antiseptic towels. Its cabin and flight crews are getting mandatory temperature checks before flights. The government recently quarantined a passenger who was later found to have the flu along with about 60 other people on the same flight who were sitting within three rows. A consultant for the microbiology division at National University Hospital in Singapore, said hygiene practices such as covering the nose and mouth when sneezing or coughing in confined areas may be the best way to limit infection and safety measures such as costly air filters may be of limited use for carriers.

Pork Products

International health officials from the CDC, WHO, FAO, OIE and other food organisations have reaffirmed that pork is safe to eat and hogs are not to blame for the epidemic. However, as of early-June, China, Russia and more than a dozen other countries were still banning pork imports from the US. This has led some US industry and government officials to "speculate that the issue is more about market share than health concerns." The bans, instituted in the wake of the swine flu outbreak, cost the US hog industry millions of dollars every week. "It's politics and not science," said John Lawrence, a professor and livestock economist at Iowa State University. "The product is safe. So why restrict imports?" About 20 per cent of US pork is exported, and China and Russia are among the biggest buyers.

In late-April, the Egyptian Government began to kill all 300,000 pigs in Egypt, despite a lack of evidence that the pigs had, or were even suspected of having, the virus. This led to clashes between pig owners and the police in Cairo. Egypt's 80-million population consisted mainly of Muslims, whose religion forbids them from eating pork, but also has an estimated 15 per cent to 20 per cent of its population being native Christians (Copts), who eat pork as part of their diet. On June 5th, the UK-based Compassion in World Farming organisation warned Egypt that its brutal measures and its mass slaughter of pigs could negatively affect Egypt's tourism industry. Philip Lymbery the chief executive of the group was quoted saying that "Britons and people from around the world have joined the international storm of protest against this atrocity in Egypt, with many saying they'll no longer consider Egypt as a possible holiday destination,"

In early-June, an Alberta Canada, a pig farmer whose herd was infected with the new swine flu virus has culled his entire herd. In May he had already culled 500 animals from his herd which was believed to have been infected by a worker who had been vacationing in Mexico. The farm owner said the animals can't be marketed because they are under quarantine and he is facing a problem with overcrowding.

Surveillance of Pig Population

At the beginning of June the US Agriculture Department said it would launch a pilot surveillance project to look for new strains of flu virus in pigs. Some experts claim that global health officials have underestimated the risk that pig herds might be a source of new influenza strains, choosing instead to focus on the threat of bird flu. "This virus most likely evolved from recent swine viruses," Gerardo Nava of the National Autonomous University of Mexico wrote in a report published in the online journal *Eurosurveillance.*

Until recently, health experts have done very little surveillance of influenza among pigs — even though the virus is very common in the animals and just as transmissible as it is among people. Flu viruses have also been shown to pass from pigs to people and from people to pigs. "These observations also reiterate the potential risk of pig populations as the source of the next influenza virus pandemic," Nava and colleagues wrote. "Although the role of swine as 'mixing vessels' for influenza A(H1N1) viruses was established more than a decade ago, it appears that the policy-makers and scientific community have underestimated it. The problem is that the virus is recombining (in the pig's body) and getting new sequences, new genes."

14

Preventive Actions

Vaccines

Influenza vaccines are typically developed to cope with seasonal flu to minimise infection rates, yet influenza still kills about 500,000 people a year around the world.

WHO recommended that vaccines for the Northern Hemisphere's 2009-2010 flu season contained an A(H1N1)-like virus. However, the version of H1N1 in the vaccine is a different, seasonal strain. Therefore, since the virus responsible for the outbreak is a new, swine-origin, non-seasonal strain of H1N1, the annual vaccination is not expected to result in human immunity.

As of mid-2009, the Communicable Disease Centre (CDC) has characterised over 80 new H1N1 viruses, all of which are related to the virus that may be used in the vaccine combatting the strain responsible for the swine flu outbreak.

Currently, most of the world's flu vaccines use an injection of "killed virus," a vaccine method made famous by Jonas Salk when he developed the first vaccine against the polio virus in 1955. As *The Economist* magazine summarised the problem, however, "if a global pandemic is declared and manufacturers are asked to produce a vaccine for [this new strain of] H1N1, they are unlikely to be able to respond quickly enough."

Furthermore, vaccine producers can produce about a billion doses of any one vaccine each year, so that even if all the capacity was switched to fight a pandemic flu, as opposed to a seasonal flu, "there would still be a huge global shortfall." Keiji Fukuda of the WHO said, "There's much greater vaccine capacity than there was a few years ago, but there is not enough vaccine capacity to instantly make vaccines for the entire world's population for influenza." The seasonal flu vaccine is not believed to protect against the new strain, therefore any existing stock would not be useful.

Production Questions and Decisions

There was also concern that should a second, deadlier wave of this new H1N1 strain appear during the Northern autumn of 2009, producing pandemic vaccines now as a precaution could turn out to be a huge waste of resources with serious results, as the vaccine might not be effective against it, and there would also be a shortage of seasonal flu vaccine available. Seasonal flu vaccine was being made as of May, according to *WebMD News*. The news site adds that although vaccine makers would be ready to switch to making a swine flu vaccine, many questions remained unanswered, including the following: "Should we really make a swine flu vaccine? Should we base a vaccine on the current virus, since flu viruses change rapidly? Vaccine against the current virus might be far less effective against a changed virus — should we wait to see if the virus changes? If vaccine production doesn't start soon, swine flu vaccine won't be ready when it's needed."

The costs of producing a vaccine also became an issue, with some US lawmakers questioning whether a new vaccine was worth the unknown benefits. Representatives Phil Gingrey and Paul Broun, for instance, were not convinced that the US should spend up to $2 billion to produce one, with Gingrey stating "We can't let all of our spending and our reaction be media-driven in responding to a panic so that we don't get Katrina. It's important because what we are talking about as we discuss the appropriateness of spending $2 billion to produce a vaccine that may never be used — that is a very important decision that our country has to make."

Moreover, should a pandemic be declared and a pandemic vaccine produced, the WHO would attempt to make sure that a substantial amount is available for the benefit of developing countries. Vaccine makers and countries with standing orders, such as the US and a number of European countries, will be asked, according to WHO officials, "to share with developing countries from the moment the first batches are ready if an H1N1 vaccine is made" for a pandemic strain. The global body stated that it wanted companies to donate at least 10 per cent of their production or offer reduced prices for poor countries that could otherwise be left without vaccines if there is a sudden surge in demand.

Gennady Onishchenko, Russia's chief doctor, said on June 2nd that swine flu is not aggressive enough to cause a worldwide pandemic, noting that the current mortality rate of confirmed cases was 1.6 per cent in Mexico and only 0.1 per cent in the United States. As a result, he stated at a press conference, "So far it is unclear if we need to use vaccines against the flu because the virus that is now circulating throughout Europe and North America does not have a pandemic nature." In his opinion, a vaccine could be produced, but said that preparing a vaccine now would be considered "practice," since the world would soon need a new vaccine against a new virus. "What's 16,000 sick people? During any flu season, some 10,000 a day become ill in Moscow alone," he said.

Production Timelines

After a meeting with the WHO on May 14, 2009, pharmaceutical companies said they were ready to begin making a swine flu vaccine. According to news reports, the WHO's experts will present recommendations to WHO Director-General Margaret Chan, who is expected to issue advice to vaccine manufacturers and the World Health

Assembly next week. WHO's Keiji Fukuda told reporters "These are enormously complicated questions, and they are not something that anyone can make in a single meeting." Most flu vaccine companies can not make both seasonal flu vaccine and pandemic flu vaccine at the same time. Production takes months and it is impossible to switch halfway through if health officials make a mistake. If the swine flu mutates, scientists aren't sure how effective a vaccine made now from the current strain will remain. Rather than wait on the WHO decision, however, some countries in Europe have decided to go ahead with early vaccine orders.

On May 20, AP reported: "Manufacturers won't be able to start making the [swine flu] vaccine until mid-July at the earliest, weeks later than previous predictions, according to an expert panel convened by WHO. It will then take months to produce the vaccine in large quantities. The swine flu virus is not growing very fast in laboratories, making it difficult for scientists to get the key ingredient they need for a vaccine, the 'seed stock' from the virus. In any case, mass producing a pandemic vaccine would be a gamble, as it would take away manufacturing capacity for the seasonal flu vaccine that kills up to 500,000 people each year. Some experts have wondered whether the world really needs a vaccine for an illness that so far appears mild."

Another option proposed by the CDC was an "earlier rollout of seasonal vaccine," according to the CDCs Dr. Daniel Jernigan. He said the CDC would work with vaccine manufacturers and experts to see if that would be possible and desirable. Flu vaccination usually starts in September in the United States and peaks in November. Some vaccine experts agree it would be better to launch a second round of vaccinations against the new H1N1 strain instead of trying to add it to the seasonal flu vaccine or replacing one of its three components with the new H1N1 virus.

The Australian company CSL said that they were developing a vaccine for the swine flu predicted that a suitable vaccine would be ready by August. However, John Sterling, Editor in Chief of *Genetic Engineering and Biotechnology News*, said on June 2nd, "It can take five or six months to come up with an entirely novel influenza vaccine. There is a great deal of hope that biotech and pharma companies might be able to have something ready sooner."

Production Capacity

US: As of 4 June, Anne Schuchat, the Immunisation Director of the CDC believed that little pandemic vaccine would be available by the fall, even if nothing goes wrong or delays production. The US goal of pandemic plans is to make 600 million doses in six months, enough for two doses for each American, according to experts, with an estimated cost of $8 billion.

Although manufacturers had a seed virus, clinical trials of their first runs would last into the summer, and federal regulators must wait until trials are finished, according to the CDC's Schuchat. Furthermore, domestic production capacity is still "completely inadequate," notes a 2008 Congressional Budget Office report, and it seemed unlikely that other nations would let vaccine factories on their soil export doses before their own needs are met.

School Closings

US: The early days of the swine flu outbreak led to numerous school closings in a number of states. However, with signs that the virus was milder than initially feared, schools reopened and the closures stopped, although officials accept that the virus is continuing to spread nationwide.

In California, school administrators have noted that throughout the US during the early weeks in the swine flu outbreak, counties recommended that schools close if a student was infected, but since early-May, as the virus spread widely across the state and country, public health experts agreed that closing schools wasn't helping contain the disease. It's not yet known whether school closings will remain relatively rare or whether more will close before summer break begins, as many schools point out that closures could become more problematic, with finals and graduations coming up.

In New York City, more than 50 public schools were closed for short periods since early-May, and as of June 5, with 780 confirmed cases in the state, the majority of cases have been mild. However, attendance dropped at other schools as worried parents kept their children home. As of early-June, a few schools were still closed. Similarly, 858 Texas schools had also closed during the outbreak with most now reopened. And in Connecticut school officials are debating the value of keeping schools closed, with 480 confirmed cases and most of them mild. There, if more than 15 per cent of the pupils had flu-like symptoms, the school would be advised to close.

Other Countries

In Australia, some schools have been closed with students and parents being advised that schools will provide schoolwork via the website, e-mail and mail. However, some school administrators have noted the major inconveniences. Trevor Gordon, principal at infected Cairns State High School, stating "We needed this like a hole in the head for our year 11 and 12 students — their exams start on June 15 and that's just six days away."

On June 6, Philippine officials announced that the start of college classes would be postponed for a week because of concerns over the rising number of swine flu cases in the country, with a reported 46 swine flu cases so far, and all with mild symptoms. The country has the most number of swine flu cases in South East Asia according to the World Health Organisation.

Containment

On April 28, WHO's Dr. Keiji Fukuda pointed out that it was too late to contain the swine flu. "Containment is not a feasible operation. Countries should now focus on mitigating the effect of the virus," he said. He therefore did not recommend closing borders or restricting travel, stating that "with the virus being widespread... closing borders or restricting travel really has very little effects in stopping the movement of this virus." However, on April 28, the US CDC began "recommending that people avoid non-essential travel to Mexico." Many other countries confirmed that inbound international passengers would be screened. Typical airport health screening involves asking passengers which countries they have visited and checking whether they feel or appear particularly unwell. Thermographic equipment was put into use at a number of airports to screen passengers. A number of countries also advised against travel to known affected regions, while experts suggested that if those infected stay at home or seek medical care, public meeting places are closed, and anti-flu medications are made widely available, then in simulations the sickness is reduced by nearly two-thirds.

Quarantines

April and May: Some countries began quarantining foreign visitors suspected of having or being in contact with others who may have been infected. In late-May, the Chinese government confined 21 US students and three teachers to their hotel rooms because a passenger on their plane to China, suspected of having swine flu, had been seated within four rows of the students. In Hong Kong, an entire hotel was quarantined with 240 guests after one person staying there was found to have swine flu.

Other governments took or threatened similar actions: The government of Australia ordered a cruise ship with 2000 passengers to stay at sea because of a swine flu threat; Egyptians who went on the annual Muslim pilgrimage to Mecca risked being quarantined upon their return.

At the end of April, when the outbreak began, Russia and Taiwan said they would quarantine visitors showing symptoms of the virus, and in Southern California, a marine confirmed to have swine flu was placed in quarantine along with about 30 other Marines. In early-May, Japan quarantined 47 airline passengers in a hotel for a week after three travellers who arrived on the same plane from Canada tested positive for H1N1 swine flu.

June: On June 8 China reported that New Orleans Mayor Ray Nagin, his wife and a security guard, although symptom free, were being held in quarantine after flying on a plane carrying a passenger who exhibited symptoms. Nagin was travelling to China and Australia on an economic development trip. However, according to Fox News, "they don't even allow phone calls," reporting that the Chinese were also screening his calls "to keep him safe," and have refused even to pass on telephone messages without the permission of government health officials.

In India, after four airline passengers from London tested positive, the government ordered that all the 231 passengers of the flight should be administered the antiviral drug Oscaltamvir. Health authorities also asked that all the passengers not move out of their homes till further orders and quarantined at least one of the infected passengers. And in Egypt, a foreign students' dormitory for the American University in Cairo, with 140 students, was put under quarantine after two US students were diagnosed with swine flu. According to the BBC, police wearing face masks "stood at barriers outside the elegant seven-floor AUC dormitory in Zamalek," and pizzas were delivered to the building during the day but none of the residents were allowed in or out.

Other governments have given health officials the "increased power" to order people into quarantine to control the spread of swine flu. The government of New Zealand, for instance, gave medical officers the power to order people to be quarantined at home if they have been in close contact with someone who has swine flu.

Planning for Emergencies

Emergency preparedness experts suggest that organisations, such as corporations, should be making plans now in case something big and unexpected happens with the

Swine Flu or other potential pandemic viruses. Kevin Nixon, an emergency planning expert who has testified before Congress and served on the Disaster Recovery Workgroup for the Office of Homeland Security, and the Federal Trade Commission, stresses that private companies "should be hammering out a game plan for who would do what and where if the government decided to restrict our movements to contain an outbreak." He states that "companies and employers that have not done so are being urged to establish a business continuity plan should the government direct state and local governments to immediately enforce their community containment plans."

Emergency planning would include some of the following: Asking people with symptoms, and members of an ill person's household, to voluntarily remain at home for up to 7 days; sending students home from school, including public and private schools as well as colleges and universities, and recommending out-of-school social distancing; and recommending social distancing of adults which could include cancelling public gatherings or changing workplace environments.

Nomenclature

Scientific Name and Common Name: According to researchers cited by *The New York Times*, "based on its genetic structure, the new virus is without question a type of swine influenza, derived originally from a strain that lived in pigs". This origin gave rise to the nomenclature "swine flu", largely used by mass media in the first days of the epidemic. Despite this origin, the current strain is a human-to-human transmitted virus, requiring no contact with swine. On April 30 the World Health Organisation stated that no pigs in any country had been determined to have the illness, but farmers remained alert due to concerns that infected humans might pass the virus to their herds. On May 2, it was announced that a carpenter on an Alberta farm who had returned from Mexico had transmitted the disease to a herd of pigs, showing that the disease can still move between species.

Debate over Name: Some authorities objected to calling the flu outbreak "swine flu". US Agriculture Secretary Tom Vilsack expressed concerns that this would lead to the misconception that pork is unsafe for consumption. The CDC began referring to it as "Novel influenza A (H1N1)". In the Netherlands, it was originally called "pig flu", then called "Mexican flu" by the national health institute and in the media. South Korea and Israel briefly considered calling it the "Mexican virus". Later, the South Korean press used "SI", short for "swine influenza". Taiwan suggested the names "H1N1 flu" or "new flu", which most local media now use. The World Organisation for Animal Health proposed the name "North American influenza". The European Commission adopted the term "novel flu virus".

After initially opposing changing the name from "swine flu", the WHO announced they would refer to the new influenza virus as Influenza A (H1N1) or "Influenza A (H1N1) virus, human", also to avoid suggestions that eating pork products carried a risk of infection. The outbreak was also called the "H1N1 influenza", "2009 H1N1 flu", or "swine-origin influenza". However, Seth Borenstein, writing for the *Associated Press* quoted several experts who objected to any name change at all.

Confirmed Cases

Dr. Jose Angel Cordova Villalobos, the federal Secretary of Health, stated on 25 April that since March, there had been over 1300 reported cases and put the death toll at 83, with 20 confirmed to be linked to a new swine influenza strain of Influenza A virus subtype H1N1. As of April 26 there have been 1,614 cases, with 103 deaths and about 400 patients in hospitals. Around two-thirds of the sick patients had recovered.

However, flu death toll in Mexico could be lower than first thought, said Dr. Gregory Evans, head of the Association of Medical Microbiology and Infectious Disease Canada and a member of a federal pandemic-planning committee, on 29 April:

There was a lot of speculation and what seemed to be evidence there were dozens and dozens of deaths. Careful analysis showed these people likely died of something else, and not flu. That's really good news, and that would fit with what we've seen outside of Mexico.

Response

After a month since the first atypical pneumonia cases were detected, the Mexican government responded and established some measures in Mexico City, the State of Mexico and the State of San Luis Potosi, where the swine flu had spread, to decrease the risk of more infections. Hundreds of soldiers and police officers mobilised by the government have handed out six million surgical masks to citizens in and around Mexico City.

On 24 April 2009, schools (from pre-school to university level) as well as libraries, museums, concerts and any public gathering place, were shut down by the government in Mexico City and the neighbouring State of Mexico to prevent the disease from spreading further; schools in Mexico City, the State of Mexico, and the state of San Luis Potosi will remain closed through at least 5 May. Marcelo Ebrard, Mexico City's mayor, has also asked all night-life facilities operators to shut down their places for ten days to prevent further infections. Health Secretary Jose Angel Cordova said on 24 April that schools will probably be suspended for at least the following week then, and that it will take around ten days to see the evolution of the virus' behaviour, and to consider other measures thereafter.

On 25 April, President Felipe Calderon declared an emergency which granted him the power to suspend public events and order quarantines. Hours later, Cordova announced classes will be officially suspended through 6 May. On 26 April, Natividad Gonzalez Paras, governor of the northeastern state of Nuevo Leon, announced that state-wide schools will remain closed until 6 May, and established a quarantine system in airports, central bus stations and the creation of observation points mainly in the southern part of the state at the nearest highways to the borders with other states, in order to realise tests conducted on people arriving from other states. Classes in Coahuila were cancelled on 27 and 28 April, with the possibility of cancelling the rest of the week. On 27 April, Health Secretary Jose Angel Cordova announced that schools of all levels throughout the nation will be suspended until May 6 in order to prevent the spread of the flu.

As part of a marketing strategy, a mascot for the outbreak was released in Mexico City on 29 April depicting a blue plush virus with black eyes in reference of H1N1; but it was discontinued two days later.

Economic Effects

The outbreak has increased the strain on an economy that was already under pressure from the current economic crisis. Although the World Bank said it would extend Mexico $25 million in loans for immediate aid and $180 million in long-term assistance, it wasn't enough to restore customer investor confidence leading to the peso's biggest tumble in six months. It seems likely now that Mexico will have to draw on a $47 billion credit line from the International Monetary Fund.

It has been reported that the food services sector within Mexico City alone is experiencing losses in the excess of $4.5 million US dollars per day. As well, it has been reported that pork meat price has dropped 30 per cent within Mexico; combined with several export bans, this will inflict severe damage to the industry. Although the virus hasn't spread throughout the whole country, as a precaution all mass gatherings have been prohibited, affecting the sports industry. Soccer teams report direct losses in the excess of $900,000 dollars per game. It also prompted cancellations of all the festivals in the country. Additionally, the Mexican race of the 2008-09 A1 GP season has had to be cancelled because of the outbreak.

15

Terminology

Phrases used to identify the flu or the causative agent include "Fujian-like" and "Fujian virus" for the H5N1 version and "Fujian-like" for the H3N2 version.

Both are also sometimes specified as "Type A Fujian flu" or "A/Fujian flu" referring to the species *Influenza A virus*. Both are also sometimes specified according to their species subtype: "Fujian Flu (H3N2)" or "Fujian Flu (H5N1)". Or both, example: "A-Fujian-H3N2".

"A/Fujian/411/2002-like (H3N2)" and "Influenza A/ Fujian/411/02(H3N2)-lineage viruses" are examples of using the full name of the virus strains.

A/Fujian (H3N2)

In the 2003-2004 flu season the influenza vaccine was produced to protect against A/Panama (H3N2), A/New Caledonia (H1N1), and B/Hong Kong. A new strain, A/Fujian (H3N2), was discovered after production of the vaccine started and vaccination gave only partial protection against this strain. Nature magazine reported that the Influenza Genome Sequencing Project, using phylogenetic analysis of 156 H3N2 genomes, "explains the appearance, during the 2003–2004 season, of the 'Fujian/411/2002'-like strain, for which the existing vaccine had limited effectiveness" as due to an epidemiologically significant reassortment. "Through a reassortment event, a minor clade provided the haemagglutinin gene that later became part of the dominant strain after the 2002-2003 season. Two of our samples, A/New York/269/2003 (H3N2) and A/New York/32/2003 (H3N2), show that this minor clade continued to circulate in the 2003-2004 season, when most other isolates were reassortants."

In January 2004, the predominant flu virus circulating in humans in Europe was influenza A/Fujian/411/2002 (H3N2)-like.

As of 15 June 2004, CDC had antigenically characterised 1,024 influenza viruses collected by US laboratories since 1 October 2003: 949 influenza A (H3N2) viruses, three influenza A (H1) viruses, one influenza A (H7N2) virus, and 71 influenza B viruses. Of the 949 influenza A (H3N2) isolates characterised, 106 (11.2%) were similar antigenically to the vaccine strain A/Panama/2007/1999 (H3N2), and 843 (88.8%) were similar to the drift variant, A/Fujian/411/2002 (H3N2).

The 2004-2005 flu season trivalent influenza vaccine for the United States contained A/New Caledonia/20/1999-like (H1N1), A/Fujian/411/2002-like (H3N2), and B/Shanghai/361/2002-like viruses.

Flu Watch reported for 13 February to 19 February 2005 that:

> "The National Microbiology Laboratory (NML) has antigenically characterised 516 influenza viruses: 470 influenza A (H3N2) and 46 influenza B viruses. Of the 470 influenza A (H3N2), 427 (91%) were A/Fujian/411/2002 (H3N2)-like and 43 (9%) A/California/7/2004-like viruses. Of the 46 influenza B, 45 were B/Shanghai/361/02-like and one B/HongKong/330/2001-like virus. Although the A/California/7/2004 (H3N2)-like isolates have reduced titres to the A/Fujian/411/2002-like antisera, the H3N2 component of the current vaccine is still expected to provide some level of protection against this new variant. The WHO has

recommended that the vaccine for the 2005/06 northern hemisphere season contain the A/California/7/2004 (H3N2)-like virus."

A/Fujian (H5N1)

Specific H5N1 isolates labelled as Fujian include A/Fujian/1/2005 and A/DK/Fujian/1734/05 (or A/Ck/Fujian/1734/2005).

A/Fujian (H5N1) bird flu is notable for its resistance to standard medical countermeasures, its rapid spread, what it tells us about the continuing evolution of the H5N1 virus, and the political controversy surrounding it. CIDRAP says "A new subtype of H5N1 avian influenza virus has become predominant in southern China over the past year, possibly through its resistance to vaccines used in poultry, and has been found in human H5N1 cases in China, according to researchers from Hong Kong and the United States. The rise of the Fujian-like strain seems to be the cause of increased poultry outbreaks and recent human cases in China, according to the team from the University of Hong Kong and St. Jude's Children's Research Hospital in Memphis. The researchers also found an overall increase of H5N1 infection in live-poultry markets in southern China."

Resistance to Countermeasures

According to the New York Times: "Poultry vaccines, made on the cheap, are not filtered and purified (like human vaccines) to remove bits of bacteria or other viruses. They usually contain whole virus, not just the haemagglutin spike that attaches to cells. Purification is far more expensive than the work in eggs, Dr. Stohr said; a modest factory for human vaccine costs $100 million, and no veterinary manufacturer is ready to build one. Also, poultry vaccines are "adjuvated" — boosted — with mineral oil, which induces a strong immune reaction but can cause inflammation and abscesses. Chicken vaccinators who have accidentally jabbed themselves have developed painful swollen fingers or even lost thumbs, doctors said. Effectiveness may also be limited. Chicken vaccines are often only vaguely similar to circulating flu strains — some contain an H5N2 strain isolated in Mexico years ago. 'With a chicken, if you use a vaccine that's only 85 per cent related, you'll get protection,' Dr. Cardona said. 'In humans, you can get a single point mutation, and a vaccine that's 99.99 per cent related won't protect you.' And they are weaker [than human vaccines]. 'Chickens are smaller and you only need to protect them for six weeks, because that's how long they live till you eat them,' said Dr. John J. Treanor, a vaccine expert at the University of Rochester. Human seasonal flu vaccines contain about 45 micrograms of antigen, while an experimental A(H5N1) vaccine contains 180. Chicken vaccines may contain less than 1 microgram. 'You have to be careful about extrapolating data from poultry to humans,' warned Dr. David E. Swayne, director of the agriculture department's Southeast Poultry Research Laboratory. 'Birds are more closely related to dinosaurs.'"

Referring to the Fujian-like strain, an October 2006 National Academy of Sciences article reports: "The development of highly pathogenic avian H5N1 influenza viruses in poultry in Eurasia accompanied with the increase in human infection in 2006 suggests that the virus has not been effectively contained and that the pandemic threat persists. Serological studies suggest that H5N1 seroconversion in market poultry is low and that vaccination may have facilitated the selection of the Fujian-like sublineage. The predominance of this virus over a large geographical region within a short period directly challenges current disease control measures." The research team tested more than 53,000 birds in southern China from July 2005 through June 2006. 2.4 per cent of the birds had H5N1, more than double the previous 0.9 per cent rate. 68 per cent them were in the new Fujian-like lineage. First detected in March 2005, it constituted 103 of 108 bird hosted isolates tested from April through June of 2006, five Chinese human hosted isolates, 16 from Hong Kong birds, and two from Laos and Malaysia birds. Chickens in southern China were found to be poorly immunised against Fujian-like viruses in comparison with other sublineages. "All the analysed Fujian-like viruses had molecular characteristics that indicated sensitivity to oseltamivir, the first-choice antiviral drug for H5N1 infection. In addition, only six of the viruses had a mutation that confers resistance to amantadine, an older antiviral drug used to treat flu."

Rapid Spread

"China's official Xinhua news agency says a new bird flu outbreak has killed more than 3,000 chickens in the northwest. The Ministry of Agriculture told Xinhua that the July 14 outbreak in Xinjiang region's Aksu city is under control. No human infections have been reported. Saturday's report says the deadly H5N1 virus killed 3,045 chickens, and nearly 357,000 more were destroyed in an emergency response. Xinhua says the local agriculture department has quarantined the infected area. The government's last reported outbreak was in the northwestern region of Ningxia earlier this month."

The October 2006 National Academy of Sciences article also says: "Updated virological and epidemiological findings from our market surveillance in southern China demonstrate that H5N1 influenza viruses continued to be panzootic in different types of poultry. Genetic and antigenic analyses revealed the emergence and predominance of a previously uncharacterised H5N1 virus sublineage (Fujian-like) in poultry since late-2005. Viruses from this sublineage gradually replaced those multiple regional distinct sublineages and caused recent human infection in China. These viruses have already transmitted to Hong Kong, Laos, Malaysia, and Thailand, resulting in a new transmission and outbreak wave in South East Asia."

H5N1 Evolution

H5N1 is an Influenza A virus subtype. Experts believe it might mutate into a form that transmits easily from person to person. If such a mutation occurs, it might remain an H5N1 subtype or could shift subtypes as did H2N2 when it evolved into the Hong Kong Flu strain of H3N2.

H5N1 has mutated through antigenic drift into dozens of highly pathogenic varieties, but all currently belonging to genotype Z of avian influenza virus H5N1. Genotype Z emerged through reassortment in 2002 from earlier highly pathogenic genotypes of H5N1 that first appeared in China in 1996 in birds and in Hong Kong in 1997 in humans. The "H5N1 viruses from human infections and the closely related avian viruses isolated in 2004 and 2005 belong to a single genotype, often referred to as genotype Z."

In July 2004, researchers led by H. Deng of the Harbin Veterinary Research Institute, Harbin, China and Professor Robert Webster of the St. Jude Children's Research Hospital, Memphis, Tennessee, reported results of experiments in which mice had been exposed to 21 isolates of confirmed H5N1 strains obtained from ducks in China between 1999 and 2002. They found "a clear temporal pattern of progressively increasing pathogenicity". Results reported by Dr. Webster in July 2005 reveal further progression toward pathogenicity in mice and longer virus shedding by ducks.

Asian lineage HPAI A(H5N1) is divided into two antigenic clades. "Clade 1 includes human and bird isolates from Vietnam, Thailand, and Cambodia and bird isolates from Laos and Malaysia. Clade 2 viruses were first identified in bird isolates from China, Indonesia, Japan, and South Korea before spreading westward to the Middle East, Europe, and Africa. The clade 2 viruses have been primarily responsible for human H5N1 infections that have occurred during late-2005 and 2006, according to WHO. Genetic analysis has identified six subclades of clade 2, three of which have a distinct geographic distribution and have been implicated in human infections:

- Subclade 1, Indonesia
- Subclade 2, Middle East, Europe, and Africa
- Subclade 3, China"

On 18 August 2006, the World Health Organisation (WHO) changed the H5N1 avian influenza strains recommended for candidate vaccines for the first time since 2004.

> "Many experts who follow the ongoing analysis of the H5N1 virus sequences are alarmed at how fast the virus is evolving into an increasingly more complex network of clades and subclades, Osterholm said. The evolving nature of the virus complicates vaccine planning. He said if an avian influenza pandemic emerges, a strain-specific vaccine will need to be developed to treat the disease. Recognition of the three new subclades means researchers face increasingly complex options about which path to take to stay ahead of the virus."

Glossary

Acute: Of abrupt onset, in reference to a disease. Acute often also connotes an illness that is of short duration, rapidly progressive, and in need of urgent care.

Airway: The path air follows to get into and out of the lungs. The mouth and nose are the normal entry and exit ports. Entering air then passes through the back of the throat (pharynx), continues through the voice box (larynx), down the trachea, and finally out the branching tubes known as bronchi.

Allergic Reaction: The hypersensitive response of the immune system of an allergic individual to a substance.

Antigenic Drift: A mechanism for variation by viruses that involves the accumulation of mutations within the antibody-binding sites so that the resulting viruses cannot be inhibited well by antibodies against previous strains making it easier for them to spread throughout a partially immune population. Antigenic drift occurs in both influenza A and influenza B viruses.

Antigenic Shift: A sudden shift in the antigenicity of a virus resulting from the recombination of the genomes of two viral strains. Antigenic shift is seen only with influenza A viruses. It results usually from the replacement of the haemagglutinin (the viral attachment protein that also mediates the entry of the virus into the cell) with a novel subtype that has not been present in human influenzaviruses for a long time. The source of these new genes is the large reservoir of influenzaviruses in waterfowl.

The consequences of the introduction of a new haemagglutinin into human viruses is usually a pandemic, or a worldwide epidemic.

Antiviral: An agent that kills a virus or that suppresses its ability to replicate and, hence, inhibits its capability to multiply and reproduce.

Asymptomatic: Without symptoms. For example, an asymptomatic infection is an infection with no symptoms.

B Virus: An infectious agent commonly found among macaque monkeys, including rhesus macaques, pig-tailed macaques, and cynomolgus monkeys. Monkeys infected with this virus usually have no or mild symptoms. In humans, however, B virus infection can result in a fatal encephalomyelitis. B virus disease in humans is extremely rare, but often fatal — an estimated 80 per cent of untreated patients die of complications associated with the infection.

Bacterial: Of or pertaining to bacteria. For example, a bacterial lung infection.

Bridge: A set of one or more false teeth supported by a metal framework, used to replace one or more missing teeth.

CDC: The Centres for Disease Control and Prevention, the US agency charged with tracking and investigating public health trends. The stated mission of the CDC is "To promote health and quality of life by preventing and controlling disease, injury, and disability." The CDC is a part of the US Public Health Services (PHS) under the Department of Health and Human Services (HHS).

Cell: The basic structural and functional unit in people and all living things. Each cell is a small container of chemicals and water wrapped in a membrane .

Centres for Disease Control and Prevention: The US agency charged with tracking and investigating public health trends. The stated mission of the Centres for Disease Control and Prevention, commonly called the CDC, is "To promote health and quality of life by preventing and controlling disease, injury, and disability."

Chemoprophylaxis: The use of a chemical agent to prevent the development of a disease.

Chills: feelings of coldness accompanied by shivering. Chills may develop after exposure to a cold environment or may accompany a fever.

Chronic: This important term in medicine comes from the Greek chronos, time and means lasting a long time.

Collateral: In anatomy, a collateral is a subordinate or accessory part. A collateral is also a side branch, as of a blood vessel or nerve.

Complication: In medicine, an additional problem that arises following a procedure, treatment or illness and is secondary to it. A complication complicates the situation.

Congestion: An abnormal or excessive accumulation of a body fluid. The term is used broadly in medicine. Examples include nasal congestion (excess mucus and secretions in the air passages of the nose) seen with a common cold and congestion of blood in the lower extremities seen with some types of heart failure.

Conjunctivitis: Inflammation of the conjunctiva, the membrane on the inner part of the eyelids and the membrane covering the white of the eye. The conjunctival membranes react to a wide range of bacteria, viruses, allergy-provoking agents, irritants and toxic agents. Viral and bacterial forms of conjunctivitis are common in childhood. Conjunctivitis is also called pinkeye and red eye.

Coronavirus: One of a group of RNA viruses, so named because they look like a corona or halo when viewed under the electron microscope. The corona or halo is due to an array of surface projections on the viral envelope.

Cough: A rapid expulsion of air from the lungs typically in order to clear the lung airways of fluids, mucus, or material. Also called tussis.

Diarrhoea: A familiar phenomenon with unusually frequent or unusually liquid bowel movements, excessive watery evacuations of fecal material. The opposite of constipation. The word "diarrhoea" with its odd spelling is a near steal from the Greek "diarrhoia" meaning "a flowing through." Plato and Aristotle may have had diarrhoia while today we have diarrhoea. There are myriad infectious and non-infectious causes of diarrhoea.

Dyspnea: Difficult or laboured breathing; shortness of breath.

Ear: The hearing organ. There are three sections of the ear, according to the anatomy textbooks. They are the outer ear (the part we see along the sides of our head behind the temples), the middle ear, and the inner ear. But in terms of function, the ear has four parts: those three and the brain. Hearing thus involves all parts of the ear as well as the auditory cortex of the brain. The external ear helps concentrate the vibrations of air on the ear drum and make it vibrate. These vibrations are transmitted by a chain of little bones in the middle ear to the inner ear. There they stimulate the fibres of the auditory nerve to transmit impulses to the brain.

Embryo: The organism in the early stages of growth and differentiation from fertilization to, in humans, the beginning of the third month of pregnancy . After that point in time, it is termed a fetus.

Epidemic: The occurrence of more cases of a disease than would be expected in a community or region during a given time period. A sudden severe outbreak of a disease such as SARS. From the Greek "epi-", "upon" + "demos", "people or population" = "epidemos" = "upon the population".

Exacerbation: A worsening. In medicine, exacerbation may refer to an increase in the severity of a disease or its signs and symptoms. For example, exacerbation of asthma is one of the serious effects of air pollution..

Fatigue: A condition characterised by a lessened capacity for work and reduced efficiency of accomplishment, usually accompanied by a feeling of weariness and tiredness. Fatigue can be acute and come on suddenly or chronic and persist.

FDA: The Food and Drug Administration, an agency within the US Public Health Service, which is a part of the Department of Health and Human Services.

Feces: The medical and scientific term for the "excrement discharged from the intestines."

Fetus: The unborn offspring from the end of the 8th week after conception (when the major structures have formed) until birth. Up until the eighth week, the developing offspring is called an embryo.

Fever: Although a fever technically is any body temperature above the normal of 98.6°F (37°C), in practice a person is usually not considered to have a significant fever until the temperature is above 100.4°F (38°C).

Flu: Short for influenza. The flu is caused by viruses that infect the respiratory tract which are divided into three types, designated A, B, and C. Most people who get the flu recover completely in 1 to 2 weeks, but some people develop serious and potentially life-threatening medical complications, such as pneumonia. Much of the illness and death caused by influenza can be prevented by annual influenza vaccination.

Food and Drug Administration: The FDA, an agency within the US Public Health Service, which is a part of the Department of Health and Human Services.

Formalin: A 37 per cent aqueous (water) solution of formaldehyde, a pungent gas, with the chemical formula HCHO, used as an antiseptic, disinfectant, and especially today as a fixative for histology (the study of tissues under the microscope).

Gastrointestinal: Adjective referring collectively to the stomach and small and large intestines.

Genetic Code: The instructions in a gene that tell the cell how to make a specific protein. A, T, G, and C are the "letters" of the DNA code. They stand for the chemicals adenine, thymine, guanine, and cytosine, respectively, that make up the nucleotide bases of DNA. Each gene's code combines the four chemicals in various ways to spell out 3-letter "words" that specify which amino acid is needed at every step in making a protein.

Genetic: Having to do with genes and genetic information.

Genome: All of the genetic information, the entire genetic complement, all of the hereditary material possessed by an organism.

Headache: A pain in the head with the pain being above the eyes or the ears, behind the head (occipital), or in the back of the upper neck. Headache, like chest pain or back ache, has many causes.

Hygiene: The science of preventive medicine and the preservation of health. From the name of Hygeia, the daughter of Asklepios, the Greek god of medicine (whose staff with entwined snake is the symbol of medicine). Asklepios (known to the Romans as Aesculapius) had a number of children including not only Hygeia but also Panaceia, the patroness of clinical medicine. Hygeia also followed her father into medicine. As the patroness of health, Hygeia was charged with providing a healthy environment to prevent illness. In Greek, "hygieia" means health.

Immune Response: Any reaction by the immune system.

Immune: Protected against infection. The Latin immunis means free, exempt.

Infection: The growth of a parasitic organism within the body. (A parasitic organism is one that lives on or in another organism and draws its nourishment therefrom). A person with an infection has another organism (a "germ") growing within him, drawing its nourishment from the person.

Influenza: The flu is caused by viruses that infect the respiratory tract which are divided into three types, designated A, B, and C. Most people who get the flu recover completely in 1 to 2 weeks, but some people develop serious and potentially life-threatening medical complications, such as pneumonia. Much of the illness and death caused by influenza can be prevented by annual influenza vaccination.

Laboratory: A place for doing tests and research procedures and preparing chemicals, etc. Although "laboratory" looks very like the Latin "laboratorium" (a place to labour, a work place), the word "laboratory" came from the Latin "elaborare" (to work out, as a problem, and with great pains), as evidenced by the Old English spelling "elaboratory" designating "a place where learned effort was applied to the solution of scientific problems."

Laser: A powerful beam of light that can produce intense heat when focused at close range. Lasers are used in medicine in microsurgery, cauterisation, for diagnostic purposes, etc. For example, lasers are employed in microsurgery to cut tissue and remove tissue.

Lungs: The lungs are a pair of breathing organs located with the chest which remove carbon dioxide from and bring oxygen to the blood. There is a right and left lung.

Mortality: A fatal outcome or, in one word, death. The word "mortality" is derived from "mortal" which came from the Latin "mors" (death). The opposite of mortality is, of course, immortality. Mortality is also quite distinct from morbidity (illness).

Mouth: 1. The upper opening of the digestive tract, beginning with the lips and containing the teeth, gums, and tongue. Foodstuffs are broken down mechanically in the mouth by chewing and saliva is added as a lubricant. Saliva contains amylase, an enzyme that digests starch. **2.** Any opening or aperture in the body. The mouth in both senses of the word is also called the os, the Latin word for an opening, or mouth. The o in os is pronounced as in hope. The genitive form of os is oris from which comes the word oral.

Myalgia: Pain in a muscle; or pain in multiple muscles. Myalgia means muscle pain. There are many specific causes of various types of myalgia. Myalgia can be temporary or chronic. Myalgia can be a result of a mild conditions, such as a virus infection, or from a more serious illness. Examples include epidemic myalgia and polymyalgia rheumatica .

Nasal: Having to do with the nose. Nasal drops are intended for the nose, not (for example) the eyes. The word "nasal" came from the Latin "nasus" meaning the nose or snout.

Nausea: Nausea, is the urge to vomit. It can be brought by many causes including, systemic illnesses, such as influenza, medications, pain, and inner ear disease. When nausea and/or vomiting are persistent, or when they are accompanied by other severe symptoms such as abdominal pain, jaundice, fever, or bleeding, a physician should be consulted.

Neurological: Having to do with the nerves or the nervous system.

NIOSH: The National Institute for Occupational Safety and Health, a US Federal agency responsible for conducting research and making recommendations for the prevention of work-related disease and injury.

Nose: The external midline projection from the face.

Onset: In medicine, the first appearance of the signs or symptoms of an illness as, for example, the onset of rheumatoid arthritis . There is always an onset to a disease but never to the return to good health. The default setting is good health.

Pandemic: An epidemic (a sudden outbreak) that becomes very widespread and affects a whole region, a continent, or the world.

Pneumonia: Inflammation of one or both lungs with consolidation. Pneumonia is frequently but not always due to infection. The infection may be bacterial, viral, fungal or parasitic. Symptoms may include fever, chills, cough with sputum production, chest pain, and shortness of breath.

Pregnancy: The state of carrying a developing embryo or fetus within the female body. This condition can be indicated by positive results on an over-the-counter urine test, and confirmed through a blood test, ultrasound, detection of fetal heartbeat, or an X-ray. Pregnancy lasts for about nine months, measured from the date of the woman's last menstrual period (LMP). It is conventionally divided into three trimesters, each roughly three months long.

Pregnant: The state of carrying a developing fetus within the body.

Prognosis: 1. The expected course of a disease .**2.** The patient's chance of recovery. The prognosis predicts the outcome of a disease and therefore the future for the patient . His prognosis is grim, for example, while hers is good.

Public Health: The approach to medicine that is concerned with the health of the community as a whole. Public health is community health. It has been said that: "Health care is vital to all of us some of the time, but public health is vital to all of us all of the time."

Quarantine: The period of isolation decreed to control the spread of infectious disease. Before the era of antibiotics, quarantine was one of the few available means for halting the spread of infectious diseases. It is still employed as needed. The list of quarantinable diseases in the US includes cholera, diphtheria, infectious tuberculosis, plague, smallpox, yellow fever, and viral haemorrhagic fevers (such as Marburg, Ebola and Congo-Crimean disease). In 2003, SARS (severe acute respiratory syndrome) was added as a quarantinable disease.

Resistance: Opposition to something, or the ability to withstand it. For example, some forms of staphylococcus are resistant to treatment with antibiotics.

Respiratory Failure: Inability of the lungs to perform their basic task of gas exchange, the transfer of oxygen from inhaled air into the blood and the transfer of carbon dioxide from the blood into exhaled air. The basis of respiratory failure may be failure of the exchange of oxygen and carbon dioxide within the tiny air sacs (alveoli) in the lungs; failure of the muscles required to expand the lungs; or failure of the brain centres controlling respiration.

Respiratory: Having to do with respiration, the exchange of oxygen and carbon dioxide. From the Latin re- (again) + spirare (to breathe) = to breathe again.

Rhinorrhea: Medical term for a runny nose. From the Greek words "rhinos" meaning "of the nose" and "rhoia" meaning "a flowing."

RNA: Short for ribonucleic acid, a nucleic acid molecule similar to DNA but containing ribose rather than deoxyribose. RNA is formed upon a DNA template. There are several classes of RNA molecules.

SARS: Severe acute respiratory syndrome. A severe form of pneumonia which appeared in outbreaks in 2003.

Sneeze: 1. As a verb, to suddenly expel air through the nose and mouth by an involuntary contraction of the muscles of expiration. 2. As a noun, the act of sneezing.

Sore Throat: Pain in the throat. Sore throat may be caused by many different causes, including inflammation of the larynx, pharynx, or tonsils.

Sore: 1. (adjective) A popular term for painful. I have sore fingers from typing dictionary terms. She has a sore throat. 2. (noun) A non-descript term for nearly any lesion of the skin or mucous membranes. He has a number of sores in his mouth.

Spanish Flu: A pandemic of influenza A (H1N1) in 1918-19 that caused the highest number of known flu deaths. More than 500,000 people died in the United States, and 20 million to 50 million people may have died worldwide. Many people died within the first few days after infection and others died of complications soon after. Nearly half of those who died were young, healthy adults. Also known as Spanish influenza.

Stage: As regards cancer, the extent of a cancer, especially whether the disease has spread from the original site to other parts of the body.

Strain: 1. An injury to a tendon or muscle resulting from overuse or trauma. 2. A hereditary tendency that originated from a common ancestor. 3. To exert maximum effort. 4. To filter.

Swine Flu: A respiratory illness of pigs caused by infection with swine influenza A virus (SIV). While swine flu viruses normally do not infect humans, occasional infections of humans do occur. Many human cases of swine influenza A virus infection occur in individuals who have had a history of recent direct contact with pigs or close (within 6 feet) contact with pigs. Rare instances of human-to-human transmission have been documented. Swine flu infections have also occurred in individuals with no history of exposure to pigs. Symptoms typically range from a mild respiratory illness to flu-like symptoms with fever. Treatment involves the use of antiviral medications begun as soon as possible after the onset of symptoms. There is no human vaccine to protect against swine flu, although vaccines are available to be given to pigs to prevent swine flu.

Symptomatic: 1. With symptoms, as a symptomatic infection. 2. Characteristic, as behaviour symptomatic of Huntington disease. 3. Directed at the symptoms, as symptomatic treatment.

Syndrome: A set of signs and symptoms that tend to occur together and which reflect the presence of a particular disease or an increased chance of developing a particular disease.

Teratogenic: Able to disturb the growth and development of an embryo or fetus.

Throat: The throat is the anterior (front) portion of the neck beginning at the back of the mouth, consisting anatomically of the pharynx and larynx . The throat contains the trachea and a portion of the esophagus .

Trimester: The nine months of pregnancy is traditionally divided into three trimesters: distinct periods of roughly three months in which different phases of fetal development take place.

Vaccination: Injection of a killed microbe in order to stimulate the immune system against the microbe, thereby preventing disease. Vaccinations, or immunisations, work by stimulating the immune system, the natural disease-fighting system of the body. The healthy immune system is able to recognise invading bacteria and viruses and produce substances (antibodies) to destroy or disable them. Immunisations prepare the immune system to ward off a disease. To immunise against viral diseases, the virus used in the vaccine has been weakened or killed. To only immunise against bacterial diseases, it is generally possible to use a small portion of the dead bacteria to stimulate the formation of antibodies against the whole bacteria. In addition to the initial immunisation process, it has been found that the effectiveness of immunisations can be improved by periodic repeat injections or "boosters".

Vaccines: Microbial preparations of killed or modified microorganisms that can stimulate an immune response in the body to prevent future infection with similar microorganisms. These preparations are usually delivered by injection.

Ventilation: The exchange of air between the lungs and the atmosphere so that oxygen can be exchanged for carbon dioxide in the alveoli (the tiny air sacs in the lungs).

Ventilator: A ventilator is a machine which mechanically assists patients in the exchange of oxygen and carbon dioxide (sometimes referred to as artificial respiration).

Viable: Capable of life. For example, a viable premature baby is one who is able to survive outside the womb.

Viral infection: Infection caused by the presence of a virus in the body. Depending on the virus and the person's state of health, various viruses can infect almost any type of body tissue, from the brain to the skin. Viral infections cannot be treated with antibiotics; in fact, in some cases the use of antibiotics makes the infection worse. The vast majority of human viral infections can be effectively fought by the body's own immune system, with a little help in the form of proper diet, hydration, and rest. As for the rest, treatment depends on the type and location of the virus, and may include antiviral or other drugs.

Viral: Of or pertaining to a virus. For example, "My daughter has a viral rash ."

Virus: A microorganism smaller than a bacteria, which cannot grow or reproduce apart from a living cell. A virus invades living cells and uses their chemical machinery to keep itself alive and to replicate itself. It may reproduce with fidelity or with errors (mutations)-this ability to mutate is responsible for the ability of some viruses to change slightly in each infected person, making treatment more difficult.

Voluntary: Done in accordance with the conscious will of the individual. The opposite of involuntary.

World Health Organisation: An agency of the United Nations established in 1948 to further international cooperation in improving health conditions. Although the World Health Organisation inherited specific tasks relating to epidemic control, quarantine measures, and drug standardisation from the Health Organisation of the League of Nations (that was set up in 1923) and from the International Office of Public Health at Paris (established in 1909), the World Health Organisation was given a broad mandate under its Constitution to promote the attainment of "the highest possible level of health" by all people. WHO defines health positively as "a state of complete physical, mental, and social well-being and not merely the absence of disease or infirmity."

Viral infection: Infection caused by the presence of a virus in the body. Depending on the virus and the person's state of health, various viruses can infect almost any type of body tissue, from the brain to the skin. Viral infections cannot be treated with antibiotics; in fact, in some cases the use of antibiotics makes the infection worse. The vast majority of human viral infections can be cured only by the body's own immune system, with a little help in the form of proper diet, hydration and rest. At times the treatment depends on the type and location of the infection and may include antiviral or other drugs.

Vital: Of a person having [illegible]

Virus: A microorganism smaller than a bacteria, which cannot grow or reproduce apart from a living cell. A virus invades living cells and uses their chemical machinery to keep itself alive and to replicate itself. It may reproduce with fidelity or with errors (mutations)—this ability to mutate is responsible for the ability of some viruses to change slightly in each infected person, making treatment more difficult.

Voluntary: Done [illegible]

World Health Organisation: An agency of the United Nations established in 1948 to further international cooperation in improving health conditions. Although the World Health Organization inherited specific tasks relating to epidemic control, quarantine measures, and drug standardization from the Health Organization of the League of Nations (set up in 1923) and the International Office of Public Health at Paris (established in 1907), the World Health Organization was given a broad mandate under its Constitution to promote the attainment of "the highest possible level of health" by all peoples. The WHO defines health positively as "a state of complete physical, mental, and social well-being and not merely the absence of disease or infirmity."

Bibliography

Alexander, D.J.: *Ecological Aspects of Influenza a Viruses in Animals and their Relationship to Human Influenza: a Review*, J R Soc Med, October 1982.

Armstrong, James F.: *Philadelphia, Nurses and the Spanish Influenza Pandemic of 1918*, Navy Medicine, March-April, 2001.

Avery, Oswald Theodore: *A Selective Medium for B. Influenzae, Oleate-hemoglobin Agar*, Journal of the American Medical Association, 1918.

Barnes, Frances M.: *Psychoses Complicating Influenza*, Missouri State Medical Association, 1919.

Bernstein, B.J.: *The Swine Flu Immunization Program*, Medical Heritage 1, 1985.

Bloomfield, Arthur, and G.A. Harrop Jr.: *Clinical Observations on Epidemic Influenza*, Johns Hopkins Hospital Bulletin, 1919.

Bogardus, F.B.: *Influenza Pneumonia Treated by Blood Transfusion*, Medical Journal, New York, 1919.

Brown, P. and Morris J.A.: *Virus of the 1918 Influenza Pandemic Era*, New Evidence about its Antigenic Character, 1969.

Bucki, Deborah: *The Other Enemy: Flu*, Buffalo Physician and Biomedical Scientist, Late Winter, Bruch, 1990.

Burnet, F.M.: *Portraits of Viruses: Influenza Virus A*, Intervirology 11, 1979.

Byerly, Carol R.: *Fever of War: The Influenza Epidemic in the US Army During World War I*, New York University Press, New York, 2005.

Chan, P.K.S.: *Pathology of Fatal Infection Associated with Avian Influenza A H5N1 Virus,* Journal of Medical Virology 63, 2001.

Charatan, F.: *UN Warns that Swine Flu Outbreak could Turn into Pandemic,* Clinical Research Ed, BMJ 2009.

Christian, Henry: *Incorrectness of Diagnosis of Death from Influenza,* Journal of the American Medical Association, 1918.

Clifford, A.B.: *Report on Influenza by the Staff, U.S. Naval Hospital, Philadelphia,* United States Naval Medical Bulletin 13, 1919.

Cohen, J. and Enserink M.: *Infectious Diseases: As Swine Flu Circles Globe,* Scientists Grapple with Basic Questions, New York, 2009.

Coker, R.: *Swine flu,* Clinical Research Ed., BMJ, 2009.

Collins, Selwyn: *Mortality from Influenza and Pneumonia in 50 Largest Cities of the United States 1910-1929,* US Government Printing Office, Washington, 1930.

Cox, Nancy J.: *Global Epidemiology of Influenza: Past and Present,* Annual Reveiw of Medicine, 2000.

Crosby, Alfred W.: *America's Forgotten Pandemic: The Influenza of 1918,* Cambridge University Press, New York, 2003.

Daer, C.C.: *The Pandemic of Influenza in 1918-19,* National Office of Vital Statistics, Washington, 1957.

Davenport, F.M.: *The Search for the Ideal Influenza Vaccine,* Postgraduate Medical Journal 55, 1979.

Davies, Pete: *The Devil's Flu: The Worlds Deadliest Influenza Epidemic,* Henry Holt & Co., New York, 2000.

Distinct, Pathogenesis: *Viruses in Mice Compared to that of other Highly Pathogenic H5 Avian Influenza Viruses,* Schultz-Cherry, Swayne, 2000.

Doty, P.: *A Retrospect of the Influenza Epidemic,* Public Health Nurse, 1919.

Douglas, R.J.: *Prophylaxis and Treatment of Influenza,* In Scientific America's Medicine, Scientific American Inc., New York, 1994.

Fauci, Anthony S.: *Pandemic Influenza Preparedness: Science and Counter Measurments,* Journal of Infectious Diseases, 2006.

Fell, Egbert: *Postinfluenzal Psychoses,* Journal of the American Medical Association 72, 1919.

Folken, F.G.: *Influenza with Unusual Complications,* United States Naval Medical Bulletin 13, 1919.

Friedlander: *The Epidemic of Influenza at Camp Sherman,* Journal of the American Medical Association 71, 1918.

Galishoff, S.: *Newark and the Great Influenza Pandemic of 1918,* Bulletin of the History of Medicine 43, 1969.

Gernhart, Gary: *A Forgotten Enemy: PHS's Fight against the 1918 Influenza Pandemic,* Public Health Reports 114, 1999.

Glezen, W.P.: *Emerging Infections: Pandemic Influenza,* Epidemiology Review, 1996.

Goodpasture, Ernest W.: *Pathology of Pneumonia Flowing Influenza,* United States Naval Medical Bulletin 13, 1919.

Hamilton, D.: *Unanswered Questions of the Spanish Flu Pandemic,* Bulletin of the American Association of the History of Nursing 34, Spring, 1992.

Hampson. A.W. and Mackenzie J.S.: *The Influenza Viruses,* Med. J. Aust. 185 (10 Suppl), November 2006.

Harrop, George A.: *The Behavior of the Blood Toward Oxygen in Influenza Infections,* Johns Hopkins Hospital Bulletin 30, 1919.

Heagerty, J.J.: *Influenza and Vaccination,* Canadian Medical Association Journal 145, 1991.

Hewer, C.L.: *1918 Influenza Epidemic,* British Medical Journal 1, 1979.

Hoagg, Jesse: *The Influenza Virus Unveiled,* The Experience, 1997.

Hoehling, A. A.: *The Great Epidemic,* Little Brown and Company, Boston, 1961.

Holland, J.J.: *The Origin and Evolution of Chicago Viruses*, Oxford University Press, New York, 1998.

Hope-Simpson, R.E.: *The Transmission of Epidemic Influenza*, Plenum Press, New York, 1992.

Hughes, Sally Smith: *The Virus: A History of the Concept*, Heinemann Educational Books Ltd., New York, 1977.

Iezzoni, Lynette: *Influenza 1918: The Worst Epidemic in American History*, TV Books, New York, 1999.

Jordan, Edwin Oakes: *Epidemic Influenza: A Survey*, American Medical Association, Chicago, 1927.

Kass, A.M.: *Infectious Diseases at the Boston City Hospital: The First 60 Years*, Clinical Infectious Disease 17, 1993.

Katz, R.S.: *Influenza 1918-1919: A Further Study in Mortality*, Bulletin of the History of Medicine 51, Winter, 1977.

Keegan, John: *The First World War*, Alfred A. Knopf, New York, 1999.

Kilbourne, E.D.: *Influenza*, Plenum Medical, New York, 1987.

King, James Joseph: *The Origin of the So-called Spanish Influenza*, Medical Record, 1918.

Kolata, Gina: *Flu: The Story of the Great Influenza Pandemic of 1918*, Straus and Giroux, New York, 1999.

Luke, Thomas, Timothy Halenkamp and Edward Kilbane: *Naval Quarantine: Impervious to Epidemics of Virulent Disease*, US Naval Institute *Proceedings* 132, New York, 2006.

MacNeal, W.J.: *Influenza Epidemic of 1918 in the AEF in France and England*, Archives of Internal Medicine, 1919.

McAnally, W.F.: *Influenza on a Naval Transport*, United States Naval Medical Bulletin 13, 1919.

McNeill, W.H.: *Plagues and Peoples*, Anchor Press, Garden City, 1976.

Microterrors: *The Complete Guide to Bacterial, Viral, and Fungal Infections that Threaten Our Health*, Tony Hart Book, 2004.

Morrisey, Carla R.: *The Influenza Epidemic of 1918*, Navy Medicine 77, 1986.

Osborn, June E.: *Influenza in America, 1918-1976: History, Science and Politics*, Prodist, New York, 1977.

Palmer, Alan: *Victory 1918*, Atlantic Monthly Press, New York, 2000.

Patterson, K. David: *Pandemic Influenza, 1700-1900: A Study in Historical Epidemiology*, Rowan & Littlefield, New Jersey, 1986.

Peters, Stephanie True: *1918 Influenza Pandemic*, Benchmark Books, New York, 2005.

Phillips, Howard and David Killingray: *Spanish Influenza Pandemic of 1918-19: New Perspectives*, Routledge, New York, 2003.

Pyle, Gerald F.: *The Diffusion of Influenza: Patterns and Paradigms*, Rowman & Littlefield, Totowa, New Jersey, 1986.

Ranger, Terence and Paul Slack: *Epidemics and Ideas: Essays on the Historical Perceptions of Pestilence*, Cambridge University Press, New York, 1992.

Reeves, R.S.: *Cholangitis Following Influenza*, United States Naval Medical Bulletin 13, New York, 1919.

Robinson, Karen R.: *The Role of Nursing in the Influenza Epidemic of 1918-1919*, Nursing Forum, 1990.

Rogers, Fred B.: *The Influenza Pandemic of 1918-1919 in the Perspective of a Half Century*, American Journal of Public Health, 1994.

Rose, H. Wickliffe: *Brittany Patrol: The Story of the Suicide Fleet*, W.W. Norton & Company, New York, 1937.

Snyder, Thomas L.: *The Great Flu Crisis at Mare Island Navy Yard*, Navy Medicine 94, California, 2003.

Stuart-Harris, C.H.: *Pandemic Influenza: An Unresolved Problem in Prevention*, Journal of Infectious Disease 122, 1970.

Sydenstricker, E.: *The Incidence of Influenza among Persons of Different Economic Status During the Epidemic of 1918*, Public Health Reports, 1931.

Tice, D.J.: *Flu Deaths Rivaled, Ran Alongside World War I*, Pioneer Planet, March, 1997.

Van, Hartesveldt and Fred R.: *The 1918-1919 Pandemic of Influenza: The Urban Impact in the Western World*, Mellen Press, New York, 1992.

Van, Reeth K.: *Avian and Swine Influenza Viruses: Our Current understanding of the Zoonotic Risk*, Vet. Res. 38 (2), 2007.

Vaughan, Warren Taylor: *Influenza: An Epidemiologic Study*, American Journal of Hygiene, Baltimore, 1921.

Watson, R.: *Swine Flu Could Come Back in More Virulent form After Summer*, European Experts Say, BMJ, 2009.

Webster, R.G., Bean W.J., Gorman O.T., Chambers T.M. Kawaoka, Y.: *Evolution and Ecology of influenza: A Viruses*, Microbiol, March 1992.

Weinstein, L.: *Influenza - 1918, A Revisit?*, New England Journal of Medicine 294, 1976.

Williams, P.M.: *High Temperature in Influenza*, United States Naval Medical Bulletin 13, 1919.

Index

I

T

V

❑❑❑